Nutrition for Runners

HILLSBORO PUBLIC LIBRARIES
Hillsboro, OR
Member of Washington County
COOPERATIVE LIBRARY SERVICES

This book has been very carefully prepared, but no responsibility is taken for the correctness of the information it contains. Neither the author nor the publisher can assume liability for any damages or injuries resulting from information contained in this book.

Jeff Galloway with Nancy Clark, MS, RD

Nutrition for Runners

Meyer & Meyer Sport

HILLSBORO PLIBRARIES
WITHDRAWN, OR
Member of Washington County
COOPERATIVE LIBRARY SERVICES

British Library Cataloguing in Publication Data
A catalogue record for this book is available from the British Library

Jeff Galloway with Nancy Clark, MS, RD: Nutrition for Runners
Maidenhead: Meyer & Meyer Sport (UK) Ltd., 2014
ISBN 978-1-78255-027-3

5416 0808 *06/14*

All rights reserved, especially the right to copy and distribute,
including the translation rights. No part of this work may be reproduced –
including by photocopy, microfilm or any other means –
processed, stored electronically, copied or distributed in any form whatsoever
without the written permission of the publisher.

© 2014 by Meyer & Meyer Sport (UK) Ltd.
Aachen, Auckland, Beirut, Budapest, Cairo, Cape Town, Dubai, Hägendorf,
Indianapolis, Maidenhead, Singapore, Sydney, Tehran, Wien
Member of the World Sport Publishers' Association (WSPA) www.w-s-p-a.org
Printed by: B.O.S.S Druck und Medien GmbH, Germany
ISBN 978-1-78255-027-3
E-Mail: info@m-m-sports.com
www.m-m-sports.com

Contents

Preface From Jeff: "Do we eat to run...or run to eat?"

Barbara Galloway and I have this debate often. The answer is...both are correct. We must accumulate the right collection of nutrients during a week of eating to restock the fuel, to repair damage, and to keep energy flowing. But it's also OK to enjoy foods and beverages. By understanding the circuits in the brain and by using the methods in this book, you can gain control over your eating and exercise.

If one of the goals is to (burn) lose fat and keep it off, Barbara Galloway and Nancy Clark offer this tip: "Give yourself a daily calorie budget." This is only one of the many contributions from Barbara Galloway to this book. Over the four decades we have been married, she has changed my diet for the better. Based upon research, and food evaluation, she uses seasonings to give wonderful flavor to vegetables, fish, and lean chicken and turkey which are the main components of our diet.

So my content in this book is actually that of Barbara and myself, and you'll find her credited in many of the chapters. I want to publicly thank her for changing my life for the better in many ways.

Introduction: Jeff's Confession: "I was a fat kid."

Like many children in Navy families, I attended 13 schools by the time I finished the 7th grade. At this point my father became a teacher, we moved to Atlanta, and my new school required each boy to exercise with an athletic team after school every day. Because of the moves, I had avoided exercise, did not have sports skills, had become lazy, and gained a lot of weight. The first few weeks were very tough and delivered a series of surprises. Even after the most exhausting workouts, I felt a boost to the attitude and spirit that I had not experienced before. The honest friendships that came from running kept me running through five years of gradual fat burnoff and modest improvement. I was hooked for life because running was transforming my brain in many positive ways. But whenever I was sidelined for a week or more due to injury, I envisioned that the fat would accumulate again. It took 20 years for this anxiety to go away.

During my first two decades of running I could find no books or guidelines on running nutrition, and I experienced about as many problems as one can have. I learned a lot about what worked best for me. But my first guru in sports nutrition was Nancy Clark. She was a marathoner in the 80's and is still a competitive runner. Her advice was based upon research and professionally guiding runners who had nutritional issues. It has been my privilege to conduct clinics with her and work on projects together. While you will find a few different interpretations of research and experience between the two of us, these issues are minor.

We want to cut through the confusing, conflicting, misinformation on running nutrition. The information we offer is based upon research and on what has worked for tens of thousands of runners.

May you run well, eat well, and enjoy both...until you are 100.

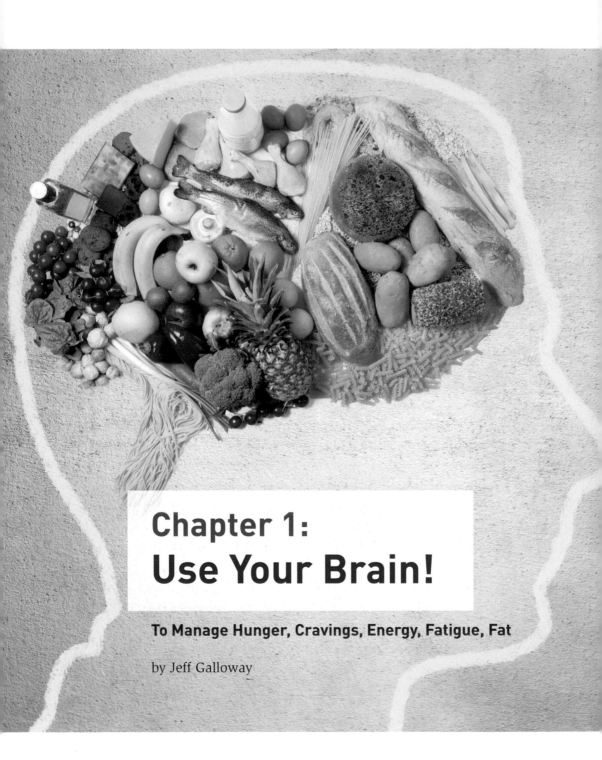

Chapter 1:
Use Your Brain!

To Manage Hunger, Cravings, Energy, Fatigue, Fat

by Jeff Galloway

© Thinkstock/iStock

As humans, we can activate our conscious brain:

- **Avoid mindless eating by managing our nutrition.**

- **Ensure we are getting adequate nutrients.**

- **Enjoy food without adding extra layers of fat.**

- **Mind and body can work together to achieve your goals.**

Average Americans today are significantly overweight or obese. I hear from many every week who tell me how dedicated I am for exercising and how they don't have the discipline to work out or eat right. My common response is "It's not really about discipline and dedication but about mentally focusing on the enrichment and pleasure that exercise brings to life." Many look at me like I'm crazy.

The fact is that all of us are capable of using our human, conscious brains to control what we do. In the process we discover far more joy throughout the mind-body network from making healthy food choices and exercising than we did eating potato chips, hot wings, etc. on the couch.

I also hear from thousands of talented runners every year who tell me that they tried to eat better but relapsed back into the "comfort foods" containing sugar, salt, and fat, which don't deliver the nutrients needed for repair and performance. Some are not overweight and some are running quite well. I tell them in the short run they may not notice a difference when they transition to healthier choices.

But I've heard from thousands who have not had the performance capacity to stay ahead of the pick-up bus in their favorite marathon or qualify for the Boston Marathon, who found that a healthy dietary change became a catalyst during their improvement journey. Because they felt better with more energy, the workouts were better—especially on the tough days. A positive change in food choices has been shown to turn on brain circuits to improve quality in exercise.

By using the simple strategies in this book you can set up a cognitive eating plan that will put you in command of your food intake and feel better every day. This can significantly improve the way you feel when running and in your daily activities. When you combine aerobic, enjoyable running with mental focus on eating, you can feel better, prepare for performance better, reduce general fatigue, and burn more fat.

We have a powerful mind-body network that is interconnected. Eating influences mental activity and mental activity influences eating—all day long. But we have many subconscious eating patterns that are deeply embedded. In this chapter I will tell you about the exciting new research that shows how you can consciously activate brain circuits to give you control over subconscious eating patterns that lower our energy and reduce motivation for running.

Yes, you can harness this network to be the master of your nutrition, feel better, improve health while controlling diet, weight, and performance nutrition.

Who's In Charge:
Conscious Brain or Subconscious Reflex Brain?

At any given moment, you can choose one of two brain operating systems: 1) the more ancient subconscious brain (SBC) located in the brainstem or 2) the conscious brain (or human brain) located in the frontal lobe.

The challenge: subconscious brain gratification eating patterns. Most humans, most of the time, allow the subconscious "reflex" brain to choose what and when to eat. This is natural because the subconscious brain (SBC) conducts most of our activities throughout the day. Hardwired in this ancient and continuously upgraded brainstem are thousands of genetically embedded and learned behavior patterns that evolved millions of years ago in response to the constant threat of starvation. To enhance survival, our SBC developed many circuits that stimulate us to eat whenever food is available and make us feel good when we eat sugar and fat. Brain circuits keep rewarding us with a "joy" hormone called dopamine even when we've eaten far more than we need for the next day or two—without feeling satisfied.

Overeating can compromise goals even for skinny runners. Even if you don't need or want to lose weight, subconscious eating patterns can cause gastro-intestinal issues that may keep you from your goals. The simple cognitive eating plans in this book can help you make the best choices before and after workouts and races so that you can perform at your best.

Use Your Conscious Brain and Gain Control Over Eating

You can take control of your nutritional destiny by having a cognitive strategy for eating (or any other activity). This shifts control out of the subconscious brain and into the frontal lobe. As you focus on what you eat, how much and when the conscious brain overrides the SBC brain. This interrupts embedded emotional subconscious eating patterns and gives you a chance to choose foods that will keep you energized and healthy, while you avoid overeating. By having an eating plan, you can combine the foods you need to balance your nutrients, keep the energy supply flowing, and avoid dehydration.

You don't have to give up the foods you love. But whether you want to ensure that you're getting the right nutrients for health and strong running, or whether you want to burn some fat, an eating strategy will allow you to achieve your goals for eating and running.

How Subconscious Brain Circuits Work

1. SBC circuits are set up to eat when food is available. Most of the energy and eating circuits were developed over millions of years ago when food was scarce and starvation was common. For survival, our appetite circuit is turned on when food is available and is not turned off until we have eaten far more than we need for that day and often the next day or two (i.e., a visit to the buffet). The extra volume not only promotes fat accumulation as a hedge against starvation, but a wealth of vitamins, minerals, and protein for repair and body function.

2. Subconscious dopamine reflex eating—no accountability. Many of the subconscious reflex brain eating patterns are not healthy or beneficial for running. Take the dopamine reflex reward pattern, for example. Dopamine is a neurotransmitter—a hormone that delivers a more powerful sense of joy than most. When you eat a food that has sugar, salt or fat, such as a potato chip (which has all three), you get a happy dose of dopamine which feels so good and is gone so fast that you reach for another and then another. If you choose to stay under the control of the subconscious brain, there is no accountability as you pile on the calories. Such eating patterns produced greater fat storage by our ancestors, which gave them a chance to make it through the weeks when food was not available. You'll find out more about this in the fat burning chapter of this book (chapter 13).

3. Stress stimulates subconscious eating patterns. Subconscious brain, when we allow it to be in control, will monitor overall stress. As stress level increases to (what it determines to be) overload, SBC will trigger the release of anxiety and negative attitude hormones. One of the most common circuits that is activated to counter this stress-negative attitude build-up is the dopamine reflex. Stress will trigger the release of negative attitude hormones. The simple subconscious fix, over millions of years, is to reach for sugar, salt, or fat and feel better quick (but only temporarily). Many runners justify "carbohydrate loading" by SBC snacking to counter the stress of an upcoming race or long run.

So it is common, when stressed or very tired, to subconsciously reach for sugary, salty, or fatty snacks to get a dose of dopamine. Unfortunately the reward is very temporary and then requires multiple doses, with no accountability. Again, the way you can gain control is to have a strategy which, will be presented in the fat burning chapter (chapter 13).

4. Damage from addictive eating patterns. Dr. Pam Peeke in her book *The Hunger Fix*, has noted the research showing how addictive eating patterns can damage the natural reward centers of the brain so that more and more junk food is needed for gratification. Ultimately there is no satisfaction and less and less dopamine when large amounts are ingested. She has also identified a detox program with exercise and eating plans that have helped thousands to enjoy eating healthy food. Here are some of the many insightful tips from this book:
   - A diet full of unhealthy fat, salt, sugar switches on certain genes to cope.
   - As one savors sugar, histones direct genes to increase insulin.
   - Increased insulin, with excess unhealthy sugar calorie intake, increases fat storage.
   - Regular, repeated insulin ingestions and secretions CAN result in insulin resistance and type 2 diabetes.
   - Too much food intake stimulates creation of fat cells.
   - Higher levels of fat trigger hormones that increase pain in joints and "weak links."

Energy is #1 Priority

Forward movement kept our ancient ancestors alive: the more territory covered, the more food gathering possibilities. Maintaining energy is top priority throughout the mind-body network, and there are many effective brain circuits that keep the energy flowing even when there are challenges.

The brain's primary fuel is blood glucose. When the supply of blood sugar is adequate, the brain will keep the many complex systems going, including an adequate energy system for muscles to do their work. If we don't eat regularly, and there is an interruption or lowering of blood sugar level, the brain will start reducing blood flow to key areas, tuning down metabolism energy level, reducing brain function, and shutting things down. Be sure to read the chapter on blood sugar maintenance.

Fat is the Back-Up Fuel

We are hardwired to store fat—for survival. Numerous internal circuits connect mind and body to ensure energy supply when food supply is below current energy needs or unavailable (periods of starvation). The brain circuit commonly called *set point* maintains and monitors fat storage and triggers an increase in appetite when set point is low and food is available. (See more in the fat burning chapter.) When on a dramatic calorie reduction, fat is released. Set point has memory, however. When one has lost 30 pounds due to a continued starvation diet, for example, and returns to eating normal levels, set point stimulates hunger a bit more, day after day, until the (before diet) set point of fat is added—often with a few additional pounds around the waistline.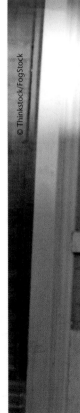

- The crucial role of regular, aerobic exercise—Your energy supply system is designed to adapt to regular aerobic exercise. Exercising about every other day will keep these circuits in good operation, while the executive brain searches for more efficient ways of eating, repairing, storing, and burning.
- In most workouts, intensity should be low so you can exercise longer and burn more calories. Workouts need to be aerobic, meaning no huffing and puffing.
- Read chapter 21, the Run-Walk-Run Method. By adjusting the amounts of running and walking, you can reduce the intensity and stress—staying in the aerobic zone.
- Gentle aerobic running stimulates production of BDNF—miracle grow for the brain and nerves, also important for memory, learning, critical thinking, and decision making

© Thinkstock/FogStock

- The meditative effect of a gentle run-walk—can help in the healing of dopamine damage from addictive eating patterns (Dr. Peeke).
- Once you burn a threshold of calories each day (usually 700-900 calories), the appetite circuit tends curb hunger.
- The satisfaction circuit.

The hunger reduction brain circuit is turned on by reaching a threshold of calories burned each day. The amount needed is between 700 and 900 calories from all sources, according to Portman and Ivy in *Hardwired for Fitness*. Gentle exercise in the morning can give you a head start on managing appetite for the rest of the day—if you are looking to lose weight and burn fat.

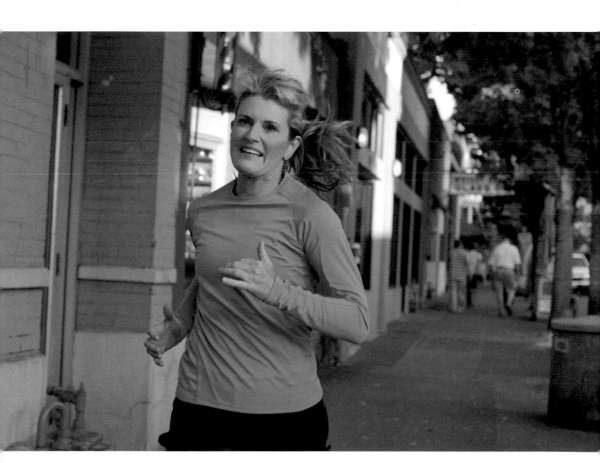

The good attitude circuit—It is well established that running activates your "good attitude" better than just about anything you can do. Run gently, turn on a good attitude, and you will be less susceptible to dopamine eating.

The vitality circuit—Thousands of runners have reported experiences similar to the following: Arriving home after a long day, I often feel too tired with, no energy to exercise. The run was scheduled but there seemed to be no resources to run for a minute or two—30 minutes seemed impossible. Promising myself that I would only go for 5 minutes, I got out the door. Surprisingly, the energy started flowing. Day after day I have to break my promise, running 30, 45, 60 minutes with no problems. Often I had more energy afterward than was experienced all day long, and did many more projects that evening than was the norm. Running at the right pace from the beginning (with the right ratio of walk breaks) activates the vitality circuit. This often reduces the craving and intake of snacks normally done to boost blood sugar on a stressful day.

The empowerment circuit—Finishing a run, especially on a tough day, turns on the empowerment circuit—which can give you the mental control to take care of your eating and your life. Running tends to activate the conscious brain which overrides the SBC. When running regularly, runners tell me that they feel more motivated to change their diet for the better. This is backed by research.

Tools That Give You Control Over Nutrition

As noted, most humans allow the emotional subconscious brain circuits to guide our eating behaviors, craving sugary, salty, and fatty foods for the temporary good feelings of a dopamine release. Other subconscious circuits are triggered to continue eating, well past nutritional needs, to store fat.

You can choose the circuits in your brain that you want to use every time you decide to eat something. Deciding will activate the conscious brain. If you have a cognitive eating strategy, you can control what goes in your mouth, maintain energy and blood sugar level, balance nutritional elements, and avoid

fat increase. This is frontal lobe eating with accountability. You are in charge!
You don't have to eat a large quantity of food to get the right balance of
nutrients—you simply need to engage your conscious brain and do the
accounting.

1. Write everything down that you eat: food, amount (ingredients if in a
   product).
2. Enter your data into a website or app.
3. Analyze your results each day or two.

All of these activate the frontal lobe so that you are in control. As you do this
regularly you will shift to conscious brain control as you consider something
to eat. Most runners who have done this, tell me that they have progressively
made healthier choices and reduced the "junk dopamine" choices.

You will learn more about how and why fat is deposited in the fat burning
section of this book. For now, realize that starvation was a major cause of
death until recent times, and there are significant brain networks to ensure
that we maintain fat levels that are usually higher than we consciously want
them to be. The fat burning section will also explain how conscious control
over eating and exercise can often help you adjust the fat level on your body.

By using the frontal lobe you can set up an eating strategy, monitor intake,
and ensure adequate intake of vitamins, minerals, and protein. In this book
you will learn the key principles in each area, with cognitive strategies. This
means that you will focus on each issue several times a day, and set up your
plan to stay on track.

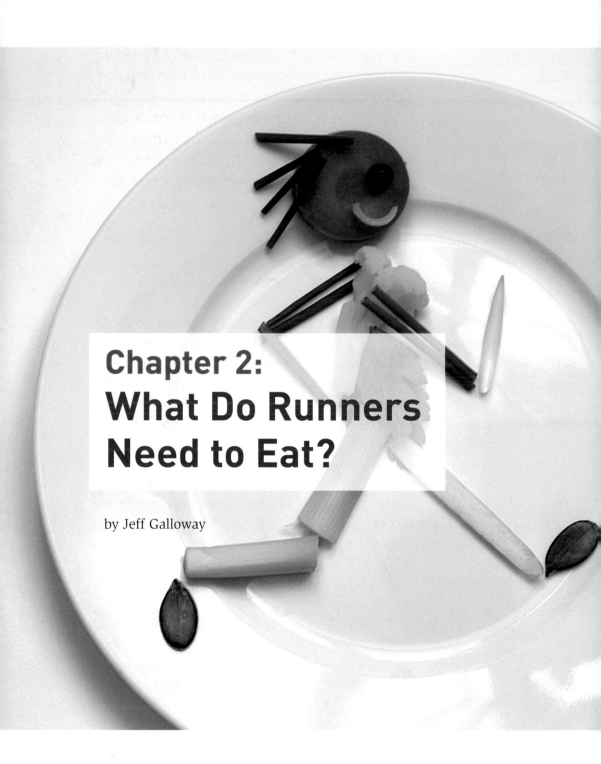

Chapter 2:
What Do Runners Need to Eat?

by Jeff Galloway

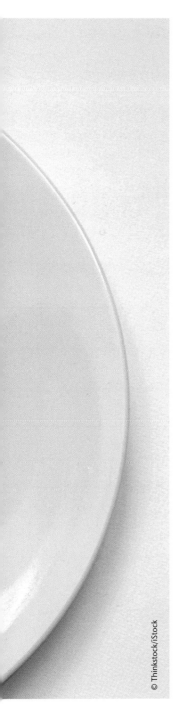

© Thinkstock/iStock

As an endurance athlete, you will not need a significant increase in vitamins, minerals, and protein. But if you don't get these ingredients for several days in a row, you will feel less energized and more tired than sedentary people. By following the guidelines below and monitoring nutrition by an app or website, you can avoid running out of gas.

Calcium, Iron, Protein

Inadequate intake of these three nutrients for an extended period can result in some serious interruption in performance. Don't worry if you miss the daily requirement of these for a day or two, you can make it up during the next few days. Here are the problems that can occur when each of these is neglected:

- Calcium is necessary for bone cell replacement and production of connective tissue and healing microtears in muscles and tendons during daily workouts.
- Iron is needed in the production of red blood cells. These transport oxygen to the muscles so they can perform.
- Protein is used in the repair and ongoing replacement of muscle cells. Runners on plant-based diets need to monitor intake and ensure that all of the amino acids are combined from the protein sources.

Carbohydrate Reloading Within 30 Minutes of Finishing

Runners often focus on loading up with a big meal before a long run or race which can cause unloading during the run. In fact, the reloading meal is much more important. If you don't reload the glycogen with a carbohydrate snack —preferably within 30 minutes of finishing a run—your muscles may not have as much bounce or capacity on the next run. Those who reload within 30 minutes of finishing a run report feeling less hungry during the rest of the day. Reload most effectively by eating within 30 minutes of finishing a run (80% carb, 20% protein). 100 calories if the run is 4 miles or less, 300 calories if the run is 13 miles or more.

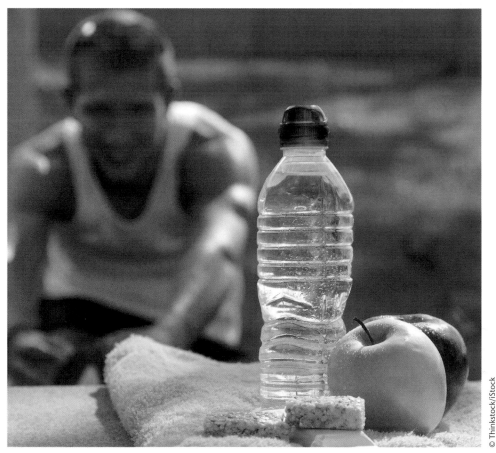

© Thinkstock/iStock

Eating a big meal the night before a morning run or race can result in unloading during the run. Use common sense during your evening meal, eating smaller portions of food that digests easily. Many runners eat a bigger meal, earlier in the day. Avoid food that tends to cause problems: high fiber foods, fatty or fried foods and any food, that has caused problems for you in the past.

Most Important Nutrient: Water
- Whether you prefer water, juice, or other fluids, drink regularly throughout the day.
- Strive for eight 8-oz (240ml) glasses.
- Caffeine drinks don't dehydrate you, so coffee and tea can count toward your fluid content, if desired.
- Alcohol has a dehydrating effect. For every glass of wine or beer, drink two glasses of water.

Drinking too much? If you have to take bathroom stops during walks or runs, you are drinking too much—either before or during the exercise. During an exercise session of 60 minutes or less, most exercisers don't need to drink at all. The intake of fluid before exercise should be arranged so that the excess fluid is eliminated before the run. Each person is a bit different, so you will have to find a routine that works for you.

My rule of thumb before long runs or races: Drink 6 oz (180ml) as soon as you wake up. That's it until you start running to avoid a lot of potty stops. There are individual differences, so practice drinking before long runs and find what works best for you.

Stomach Issues During Long Runs or Races

Those who have upset stomachs or many bathroom stops during long runs or races should watch the quantity of food eaten the afternoon and evening (day before) and the morning of the run. Practice eating the day before each long run and journal what, how much, and when. Fine-tune this through the training season and use the successful plan the day before your race. Limit fat, high fiber foods, and think twice before eating large portions of meat or large portions of any food for that matter.

Sweat the Electrolytes

Electrolytes are the salts that your body loses when you sweat: sodium, potassium, magnesium, and calcium. When these minerals get too low, your fluid transfer system doesn't work as well, and you may experience ineffective cooling, swelling of the hands, and other problems. Most runners have no problem replacing these in a normal diet, but if you are regularly experiencing cramping during or after exercise, you may be low in sodium and fluids, but might also just have tired but hyper-active muscles that cramp, unrelated to nutrition.

Practical Eating Issues

- Most of my runners who have had stomach issues, have found that they did not need to eat as much before a run. Exceptions are diabetics and those with severe hypoglycemia. See the next chapter.
- The standard recommendation is 2 calories per pound bodyweight (or adjusted bodyweight) within 5 to 60 minutes pre-exercise, but most of the novice runners I've coached who consume this much before a run have digestive problems.
- During long runs and races, my rule of thumb is 2-4 oz of water, every two miles (60-120 ml). Among my runners there has been a high percentage of nausea issues when drinking electrolyte beverages.
- My blood sugar booster rule of thumb during long runs and races is 30 to 40 calories every two miles. Use various snacks during long runs to find the one that works best for you; gummi bears, hard candy, gels, energy bars, and sugar cubes have produced the least number of stomach issues among my runners.

- If you are running low on blood sugar at the end of your long runs, increase your blood sugar booster snacks from the beginning of your next run (see the next chapter for more information).
- It is rarely a good idea to eat a huge meal—especially the night before a long run or a race. Those who claim that they must "carbo load" with a large meal the night before are most likely rationalizing their desire to eat a lot of food. For many runners, eating a big meal the night before a long run can result in unloading during the run.

Jeff's Suggested Long Run or Long Race Eating Schedule
- As soon as you awaken drink either a cup of coffee or a 6-oz glass of water (180 ml).
- 30 minutes or less before any run (if blood sugar is low): approximately 100 calories of a blood sugar booster snack. (If blood sugar is OK, there is no need to consume this snack. The standard recommendation is 2 calories per pound bodyweight within 5 to 60 minutes pre-exercise. Find what works for you.
- Within 30 minutes after a long run: approximately 100-300 calories of a 80% carb, 20% protein

Hint: Caffeine, when consumed before exercise, engages the systems that enhance running and extend endurance—and caffeine does not cause dehydration.

Eating and Drinking Before an Evening Event

To ensure the best experience when running at night, you need to focus on what to eat before running at night, and practice. With proper scheduling of your snacks, leading up to the race you can maintain a good blood sugar level while avoiding nausea from eating too much.

An eating plan. Gain control over your energy level and your digestive issues by developing and testing an eating plan, during the five hours before the race. Here are my suggestions, based on the eating success of many runners under similar situations:

- Morning: Eat somewhat normally but avoid large meals.
- Afternoon: Consume light snacks of 150-250 calories, about every two hours, with 4-6 oz of water.
- The standard recommendation is 2 calories per pound bodyweight (or adjusted bodyweight) within 5 to 60 minutes pre-exercise—find what works for you.
- Evening: Most find it best to stop eating two hours before the run. Adjust to your needs. If your blood sugar starts to drop, have a light snack, such as an energy bar or gummi bears, Superfruit bits (no more than 150 calories, 30 minutes before the race).
- Avoid snacks that are high in fat, or high in fiber. Choose foods that are easy to digest.
- Drink 4-6 oz of water with each snack.
- Blood sugar insurance. Carry a baggie of blood sugar booster snacks such as gummi bears, hard candies, Superfruit bits, sugar cubes, or the sugar source of your choice, during the half hour before the start.
- Blood sugar boost during the long runs or race. My rule of thumb is 30-40 calories every two miles. Nancy Clark notes that the consensus among sports medicine and sports nutrition professionals for all sports is this: 120-240 calories of carbohydrate (30-40 g) for exercise that lasts 1-2.5 hours, and 240-360 calories of carbohydrate (60-90 g) for exercise that lasts for more than 2.5 hours.

Try this and fine-tune it to your needs. Bring a baggie of the snacks that you have used successfully, and you can maintain control over low blood sugar.

Fluids:

- Morning: Drink 6-8 oz of fluid every hour. One 8-oz drink could be an electrolyte beverage, but standard foods are the better source of carbohydrates.
- Afternoon: Drink 4-6 oz of fluid every hour.
- Drink 4-6 oz of fluid with each snack.
- During the two hours before long runs or races, it's best to stop drinking or

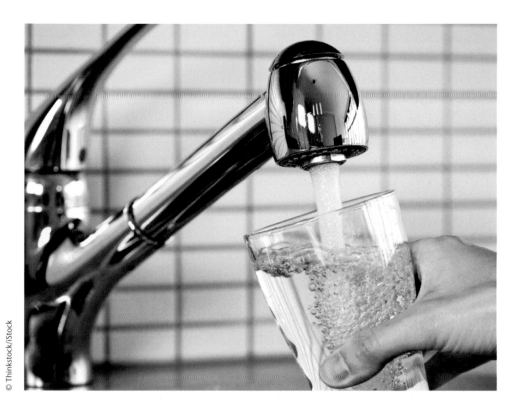

© Thinkstock/iStock

minimize fluid intake (so that you can take your potty stop before the start of the run, instead of during the run).

- Avoid alcohol before the race.
- Caffeine is generally OK if you are used to consuming it before runs. Generally it's best to drink your last caffeinated beverage about two hours before the start—but do what works for you.
- The rule of thumb during the race is 2-4 oz of water every two miles or according to thirst. Don't drink more than 20 oz an hour.
- Enjoy every mile and the party afterward.

Practice running and eating in the evening.
During the training period, schedule at least two of your runs at about the time the race will start. This will help you adjust to running at night. Even more important, journal your eating leading up to the night run. Adjust intake as needed.

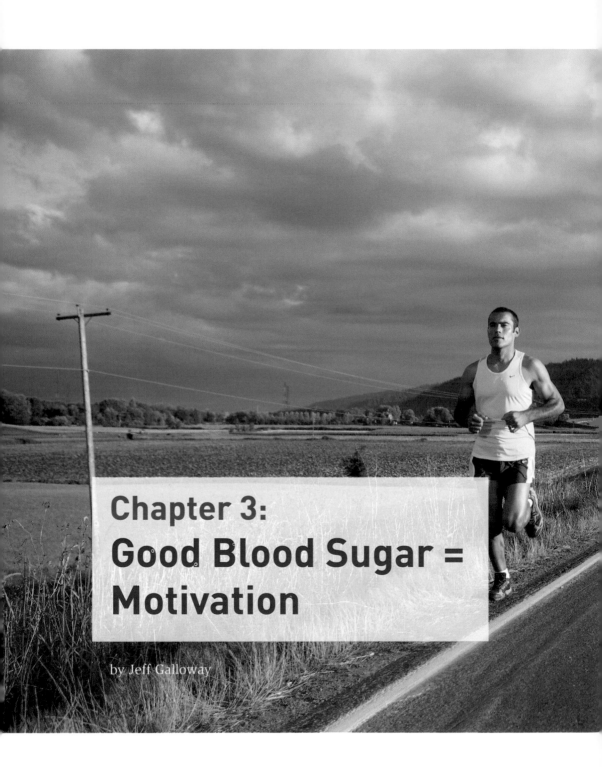

Chapter 3:
Good Blood Sugar = Motivation

by Jeff Galloway

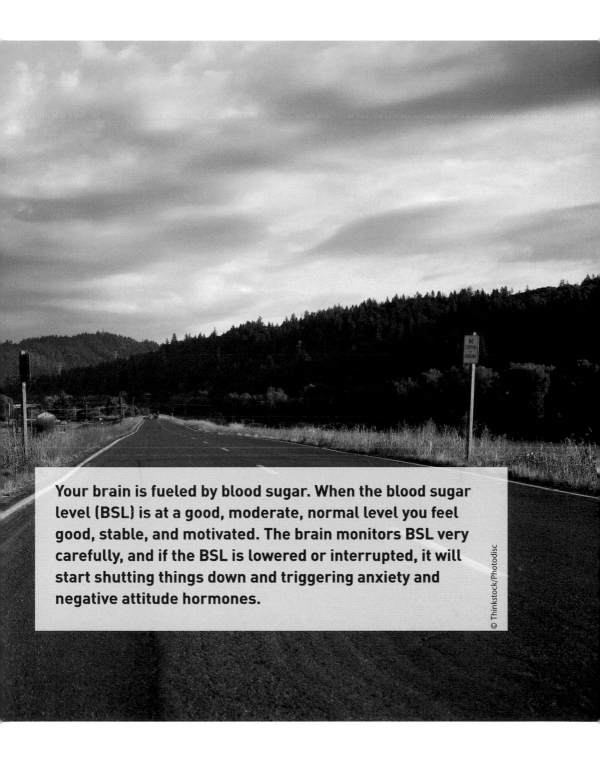

Your brain is fueled by blood sugar. When the blood sugar level (BSL) is at a good, moderate, normal level you feel good, stable, and motivated. The brain monitors BSL very carefully, and if the BSL is lowered or interrupted, it will start shutting things down and triggering anxiety and negative attitude hormones.

© Thinkstock/Photodisc

Some runners I've coached find that if they eat too much sugar, 45 or more minutes before a run, the BSL can rise too high. You'll feel really good for a short period, but the excess sugar triggers a release of insulin. This reduces BSL—to an uncomfortable level. In this state your energy drops, mental focus is foggy, and motivation goes down rapidly.

When blood sugar level is maintained throughout the day, you will be more motivated to exercise, add other movement to your life, be mentally active, deal with stress, and solve problems. Just as eating throughout the day keeps metabolism up, the steady infusion of balanced nutrients all day long will maintain stable BSL. This produces a feeling of well-being.

You don't want to get on the "bad side" of your BSL. Low levels are a stress on the brain—literally messing with your mind. If you have not eaten for several hours before a run-walk, and BSL drops, you'll receive an increase in the number of negative and anxiety hormones, reducing motivation to exercise.

The simple act of eating about 100 calories within 30 minutes before running, can reduce the negative, make you feel good, and get you out the door. This can be the difference in whether you run, or not. The standard recommendation is 2 calories per pound bodyweight within 5-60 minutes pre-exercise. Find out what works best for you.

The BSL Roller Coaster

Eating a snack with too many calories of simple carbohydrate can be counter-productive for BSL maintenance. As mentioned above, when the sugar level gets too high, your body produces insulin, sending BSL lower than before. The tendency is to eat again, which produces excess calories that are converted into fat. But if you don't eat, you'll stay hungry and pretty miserable—in no mood to exercise or move around and burn calories or get in your run for the day. A simple solution is to eat grains instead of simple sugars or combine protein with carbs.

Try Eating Every 2-3 Hours

Once it is established which snacks work best to maintain your BSL, most runners maintain a stable blood sugar level by eating small meals regularly, every 2-3 hours. As noted in the previous chapter, it's best to combine grains, fruits, and vegetables with protein and a small amount of fat.

Do I have to eat before running?

Only if your blood sugar is low. Most who run in the morning don't need to eat anything before the start if there was adequate food consumption the day before. But for many active people, blood sugar drops overnight and they feel better and run better with a pre-run snack. As already mentioned, if your blood sugar level is low in the afternoon, and you have a run scheduled, a snack can help when taken about 30 minutes before the run. If you feel that a morning snack will help, the only issue is to avoid consuming so much that you get an upset stomach.

Eating During Exercise

Most exercisers don't need to worry about eating or drinking during a run until the length exceeds 90 minutes as long as they have had adequate pre-exercise fuel. At this point, there are several options. In this case, most runners wait until the 30- to 40-minute mark in the workout before starting to take the blood sugar level (BSL) booster. Diabetics may need to eat sooner and more often—but this is an individual issue.

The brain's fuel is blood glucose. If you don't keep this boosted during a long run, the brain will be deprived and will start shutting things down. Avoid this by trying different snacks and using the one that works best for you.

Jeff's Rule of Thumb: Consume 30-40 calories about every two miles (20-25 minutes), with 2-4 oz of water (60-120 ml).

Easiest to digest:
- Candy—particularly gummi bears or hard candies, such as lifesavers.
- Sugar Cubes or tablets—this is the simplest of the BSL booster snacks, and the easiest on the stomach for most runners.
- Superfruit—an all-fruit snack in bits and has worked well for many of my runners, including me (I am helping to promote this no-additive natural product but receive no fee for doing this). While any dried fruit can work, many runners I've heard from have problems with dried fruit who don't have problems with Superfruit.

Other products:
- Energy Bars—cut into small pieces. Avoid products with a lot of fiber, fat, or protein.

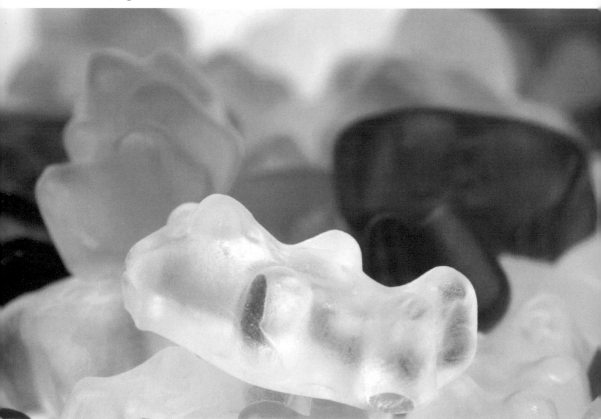

- Gel products—these come in small packets, and are the consistency of honey or thick syrup. The most successful way to take them is to put one to three packets in a small plastic bottle with a pop-top. About every 10-15 minutes, take a small amount with a sip or two of water. Many runners report nausea at the end of races when using this type of product.
- Sports drinks—I've noticed that a significant percentage of my runners who drink sports drinks during a run experience nausea. If you have found this to work for you, use it exactly as you have used it before.

Reloading 100-300 Calories Within 30 Minutes After Exercise

© Thinkstock/iStock

Whenever you have finished a hard or long workout, a recovery snack can help you recover faster. Again, the 80:20 ratio of simple carbohydrate to protein has been most successful in reloading the muscles.

Nancy Clark suggests that instead of getting caught up in ratios, you can simply enjoy recovery foods of choice: primarily carbohydrate with a little protein, such as chocolate milk, flavored yogurt, eggs and toast, cereal with (soy) milk, a sandwich, pasta with meat sauce, beans, and rice.

Many of my runners feel bloated if they eat regular food immediately after a long or hard run and don't have problems with simple carbs.

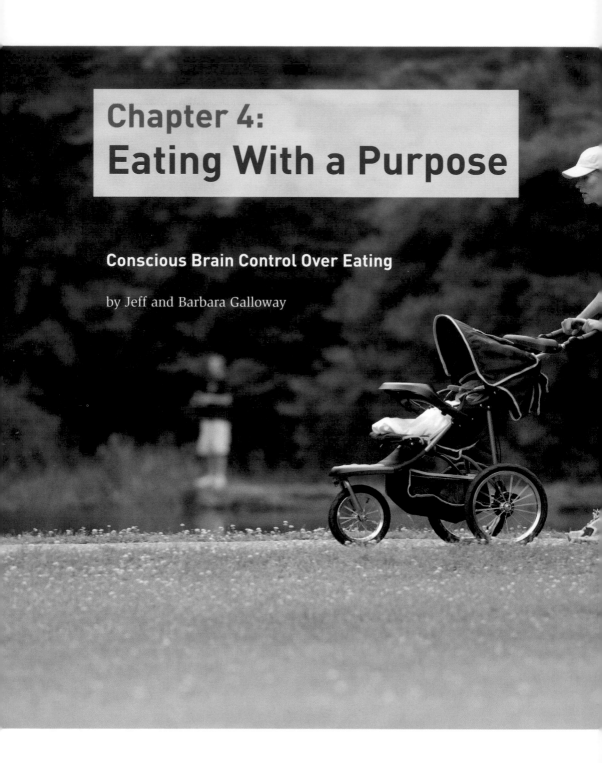

Chapter 4:
Eating With a Purpose

Conscious Brain Control Over Eating

by Jeff and Barbara Galloway

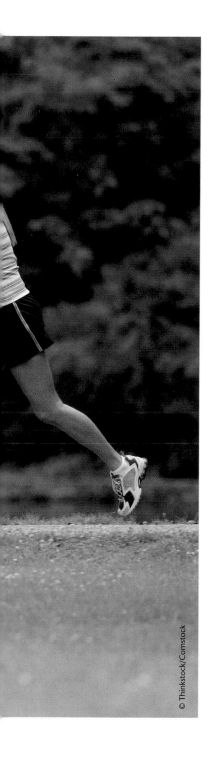

© Thinkstock/Comstock

- Know the calorie content and nutrient breakdown of what you're eating (read the label or use a website like www.fitday.com).
- Concentrate on the positive: "I can eat more of (good tasting fruit and crunchy vegetables) rather than "I have to eat less of _____.""
- Visualize the food on your plate as being in your stomach. Ask yourself, "Do I want to stretch my stomach to cram in more food?" "Do I need that much right now?"
- Don't have more than three items or dishes at one meal.
- Drink a glass of water (6-8 oz) before eating, and drink 4-6 oz during the meal.
- Hot fluids (tea, coffee, broth) leave you feeling more full than cold fluids.
- Never eat fatty appetizers if you are very hungry before a meal. Instead, choose soup, salad, hot tea or warm skim milk.
- Take vitamins with a meal and avoid caffeine for half an hour.
- Don't even think about going to a buffet.
- Visit the grocery store with a mission. Have a list of exactly what you will buy and only buy what is on the list.
- Veggies: steam, toast, or stir-fry—or eat them raw or in salads.
- Use nonfat dressings or spray-on dressings for salads.
- Eat slowly! Increase the number of chews for each bite—this triggers more satisfaction in the stomach.

- Count every calorie eaten—it only hurts you to "forget" the amount or certain foods in your totals.
- Fluid calories add up quickly. Budget your alcohol, fruit juice, and other fluids.
- Buy the highest quality foods: lean meats, fruits, veggies, and whole grain products. These may cost a little more but you'll appreciate the quality, especially when the taste is better. You will feel better about the quality of your nutrition.
- Herbs and spices can enhance the savory flavor of foods, leaving you satisfied with fewer calories consumed.
- Try to accumulate your daily quota of vitamins and minerals from food. If your daily analysis of nutrients shows regular deficiencies (based upon the recommended daily allowance, RDA) then find a really good vitamin. Jeff travels a lot and takes Cooper Complete vitamins, designed by Dr. Kenneth Cooper. No vitamin pill can compensate for an inadequate diet.
- In choosing a restaurant, check out the websites to find one that breaks down the nutritional composition of the menu items. By planning ahead, you can avoid impulsive dopamine gratification eating.
- Another option is to get a nutritional guide when you arrive at the restaurant and analyze it before the waiter takes your order.
- Try to avoid or severely limit trans fat and saturated fat. Use olive oil or eat fish that have omega-3 fat (usually cold water species).

Focused Eating

Letting the conscious brain make the decisions
- Focusing on each food choice activates the conscious brain.
- This gives you control over your nutrition.
- You assume responsibility for your eating and your exercise.
- Don't give up if you have a bad day—account for it and go on.
- Enjoyment of exercise turns on many nutritional circuits.
- You are in command of a calorie budget, as you add gentle movement to your daily activities.

Part one: Eating with a purpose. We want you to choose food that is easily available, most of which can be prepared quickly. You'll see how to set up your eating plan to gain control over the calorie balance each day, as well as the vitamins, minerals, and other nutritional ingredients you need each day. Websites are great tools because you'll learn portion control—while you account for needed nutrients. You'll also learn whether you're getting the nutrients you need and then adjust with an eating plan to compensate if needed. Staying focused on the purpose keeps you in the frontal lobe.

Part two: Creating your fat-burning furnace. By gradually increasing a long run, you will train thousands of muscle cells to burn more fat—not only while exercising. Once adapted to fat burning, these muscle cells will burn more fat when you're sitting and walking around—even at night when asleep! But take note: to lose fat you need to create a calorie deficit. Burning fat does not equate to losing body fat.

Part three: Taking more steps per day. Get a step counter and increase the number of steps taken per day. As you do your daily activities, fill up the "dead time" when you would be sitting by walking segments of 5-10 minutes at a time. Extra steps, in segments of 500-2,000 do not tend to increase appetite—but they burn fat all day long.

A Positive Relationship With Food

A cognitive approach to food intake is crucial for weight loss, replacing nutrients, and recovery.

- A negative relationship means subconscious eating to make you feel better.
- A positive relationship means managing your food choices so that you have energy all day long.
- Each day you have a budget of calories—ensuring accountability.
- Energy is maintained by eating more often: six to eight times a day—schedule these and prepare.

- Focus on each food choice, choosing snacks that leave you satisfied because nutrients are balanced.
- Each snack has a purpose—it's important to get calcium, iron, and protein.
- Variety is important. Even if you really like a snack don't eat it all day long, day after day.
- You can still eat and drink some favorites (decadent choices), but they must be budgeted.
- You are in control, your conscious brain is in control, and you feel good.

Two Burning Issues When Losing Fat

Fat burning, not weight loss: While the scales are an important tool, you cannot be obsessed about daily changes in weight. Fluid fluctuations in your body will have you up one day, down the next. As you adjust your daily exertions and smaller but energizing meals, you can control the process through real fat burnoff. The scales will continue to fluctuate somewhat, but the overall fat level can be reduced—even if the "daily scales report" is a bit higher on some days. Stay focused on the long term average weight.

Good weight vs bad weight: Muscle mass that is used during exercise, regularly, weighs more than an equivalent mass of untrained muscle fibers. Beginners often experience a slight weight gain as the muscle adapts in many ways: extra storage for fuel, more water for cooling off and processing energy, and increased blood volume for delivery of oxygen and withdrawal of waste products. Your muscles are being transformed into vibrant athletic muscles that can burn a lot of fat often with less fatigue than you are experiencing now.

YOU can enjoy food that is healthy and energizing. If you don't like certain items now, combine them with other foods and use some of the great seasoning combinations in recipes from publications such as *Cooking Light* magazine. You can learn to like almost anything—and feel better for doing so. To feel good and to maintain a high level of health, you need to eat foods every day that are nutritionally balanced.

YOU have an amazing ability to use the brain to control the stomach. Unfortunately this is usually done during crash diets that set up negative after-effects. We can just as easily program ourselves to eat energizing food, frequently throughout the day, in quantities that don't add fat to our bodies.

YOU can budget calories. Women have to handle budgets constantly—and budgeting means putting the conscious brain in control, reducing the chance of subconscious dopamine eating. You can still eat the chocolate or have a glass of wine, but you must adjust for them in your budget. You determine how you will consume your allocation, each day.

YOU can change your relationship with food in a positive direction. You may use food now to drown sorrows deal with stress or disappointments. But once you realize that this is a bad relationship which you must exit, you are open to a positive one: eating every two to three hours, feeling good, and finding new foods that you like.

YOU can be in control of the situation. By using your executive brain in the frontal lobe, you can stay focused on food all day and use a "reality check" nutritional website to stay on track.

Changing the relationship can be stressful. Gentle exercise is a powerful tool that can erase and manage an amazing amount of stress. Realize that there will be tough times and don't give up. Millions of runners have made the shift and feel so much better. But unconscious stress build-up can trigger aches and pains and magnify them. To understand this process and manage it, we recommend using the method in two breakthrough books: *Mental Training for Runners: How to Stay Motivated* by Jeff and Barabara Galloway, and *The Mindbody Prescription* by Dr. John Sarno.

YOU can feel better. Once the relationship is working, you feel better throughout the day because you're in control. Reinforce this good feeling by recognizing that your efforts are making a difference. Some runners reward themselves at this point with a new outfit—one size down.

Key Principles:

- Crucial: Control calorie intake and let exercise contribute to a calorie deficit (so your exercise can burn off the fat).

- Food is fuel for the next workout or the next three hours—keep it flowing in controlled amounts.

- Food contains the building blocks for muscle, bone, and organs and must be replaced daily.

- Budget daily totals through portion control.

- Combine foods so that you feel satisfied with fewer calories consumed.

- Get a "reality check" as you account for the calories every night—eaten and burned (vitamins, minerals, protein).

- You're in control: Set up your reality check—websites, apps, weight monitoring programs.

- The key to feeling good is managing blood sugar level, which helps you maintain motivation.

- Eat every two to three hours.

- Never say never—don't totally abstain from foods you love, ration them.

- Drink water or other low- or non-calorie drinks with food and throughout the day to feel satisfied longer.

- Crucial for workout energy: Eat 100-300 calories within 30 minutes of finishing a workout (composed of 80% simple carb, 20% protein).

More energy to exercise. If you're eating regularly, you will have more energy to do everything, including exercise, by adding more steps to your day.

Final Thoughts

- Sally dieted and lost over 70 pounds in six months, but gained back more than that amount within a year.
- Elaine, who exercised and ate mindfully, lost 98 pounds and kept it off, five years and counting. She learned to enjoy exercise, and, along with her new eating habits, the exercise helped keep the weight from being deposited again.
- Starvation diets show a water weight loss which is quickly added back.
- The exercise-good food relationship creates a behavioral change—you feel good.
- Snacking is OK! But you must choose the right snacks.
- Gain control over the intake side by using one of many good websites. I use www.fitday.com.
- A suggested eating schedule will be offered in this book.

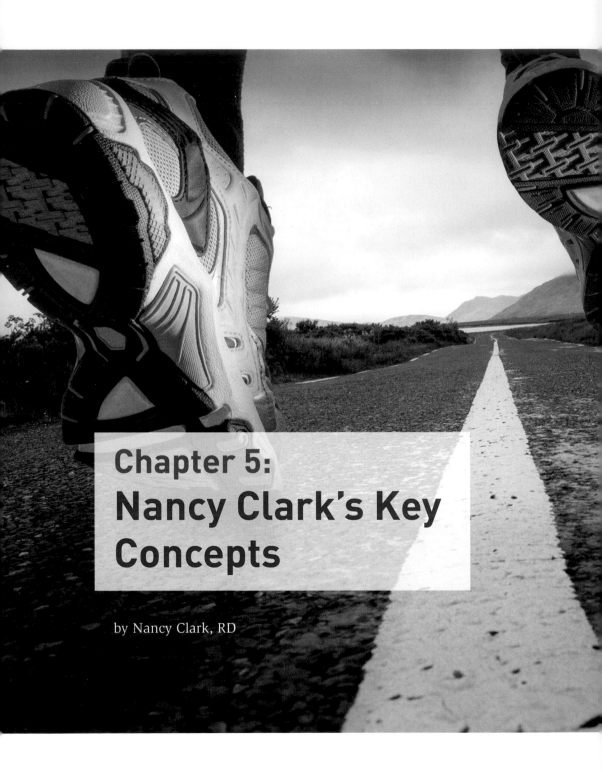

Chapter 5:
Nancy Clark's Key Concepts

by Nancy Clark, RD

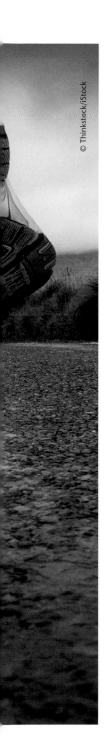

© Thinkstock/iStock

Fueling yourself well on a daily basis requires time management skills. You need to learn how to manage to find time to:

- **food shop so you'll have wholesome sports foods available.**

- **fuel up and refuel at the right times.**

In this chapter, I'll share with you the basic tips about how to eat well, even when you are eating on the run and even if you are not much of a cook. But first, it helps to understand my definition of "eating well."

My simple definition is to–
1. Eat at least three kinds of wholesome foods at each meal.
2. Eat two kinds of wholesome foods at each snack.
3. Eat on a time line—even—sized meals throughout the day, as opposed to crescendo-eating (a small breakfast and a belly-stuffing meal at the end of the day).
4. Choose to eat at least 90% of the calories from quality foods and, if desired, the remaining 10% from sweets and treats.

Some Top Sports Foods
Many marathoners don't have time to cook or prepare foods. Here are some readily available, ready-to-eat, nutrient-dense sports foods to help you easily enjoy a top sports diet.

Some of the best fruits for vitamins A and C:
Oranges, grapefruit, mangos, bananas, melons, berries, kiwi

Some of the best vegetables for vitamins A and C:
Broccoli, spinach, green and red peppers, tomatoes, carrots, sweet potato, winter squash

Easy sources of calcium for strong bones:
Low-fat milk, yogurt, cheese, calcium-fortified orange juice, soy milk, and tofu

Convenient pre-cooked (or no-cook) proteins for building and protecting muscles:
Deli roast beef, ham, and turkey; canned tuna and salmon; hummus; peanut butter; tofu; cottage cheese; canned beans (pinto, kidney, garbanzo)

Cook-free grains for carbohydrates and fiber:
High-fiber breakfast cereals (preferably iron-enriched), wholesome breads and bagels, whole-grain crackers

Take Note: You don't have to be a good cook to eat well. You just need to be a smart shopper. I'll help you with that!

To help guide optimal food choices, many countries and health organizations have created dietary guidelines. The guidelines for the US describe a healthy diet as one that emphasizes fruits, vegetables, whole grains, and fat-free or low-fat milk and milk products; includes lean meats, poultry, fish, beans, eggs, and nuts; and is low in saturated fats, trans fats, cholesterol, salt (sodium), and added sugars. More specifically, this is what you want to keep in mind as you make your daily food choices:

- Try to eat at least 2 cups of fruit and 2 1/2 cups of vegetables per day. (This is the reference for a 2,000-calorie intake; most runners need more calories than that and could wisely consume some of those extra calories from fruits and vegetables.)
- Choose a variety of colors of fruits and vegetables each day: red apples, green peppers, orange carrots, white potatoes.
- Enjoy whole-grain products at least two times per day, such as oatmeal for breakfast and whole-wheat bread for lunch. The rest of the recommended grains can come from enriched grain products, such as enriched pasta. In general, at least half the grains should come from whole grains. (Whole grains include wheat, rice, oats, corn, and barley.)

• Drink 24 ounces (3 cups; 720 ml) per day of fat-free or low-fat milk or
  yogurt, or the calcium-equivalent in low-fat cheese (8 oz of milk or yogurt
  = 240 ml = 1 cup = .75 ounces [20 g] of cheese).

Dietary Recommendations for Good Health

By following these dietary recommendations, you can substantially reduce
your risk of developing heart disease and other diseases of aging.
• Balance calorie intake and physical activity to achieve and maintain a
  healthy body weight.
• Consume a diet rich in vegetables and fruits.
• Choose whole-grain, high-fiber foods.
• Consume fish, especially oily fish, at least twice a week.
• Limit your intake of saturated fat to < 7% of energy, trans fat to < 1% of
  energy, and cholesterol to < 300 mg per day by
    • choosing lean meats and vegetable alternatives,
    • selecting fat-free (skim), 1%-fat, and low-fat dairy products,
    • minimizing intake of partially hydrogenated fats.
• Minimize your intake of beverages and foods with added sugars.
• Choose and prepare foods with little or no salt.
• If you consume alcohol, do so in moderation.
• When you eat food that is prepared outside of the home, follow these
  dietary recommendations.
• When selecting and preparing meat, poultry, dry beans, and milk or milk
  products, make choices that are lean, low-fat, or fat-free.
• Limit your intake of saturated and trans fats and choose healthier oils such
  as olive and canola oils, nuts and nut butters, and oily fish such as salmon.

*Source: Diet and Lifestyle Recommendation Revision 2006: A Scientific
Statement From the American Heart Association Nutrition Committee. A.
Lichtenstein et al. Circulation 2006; 114:82-96.*

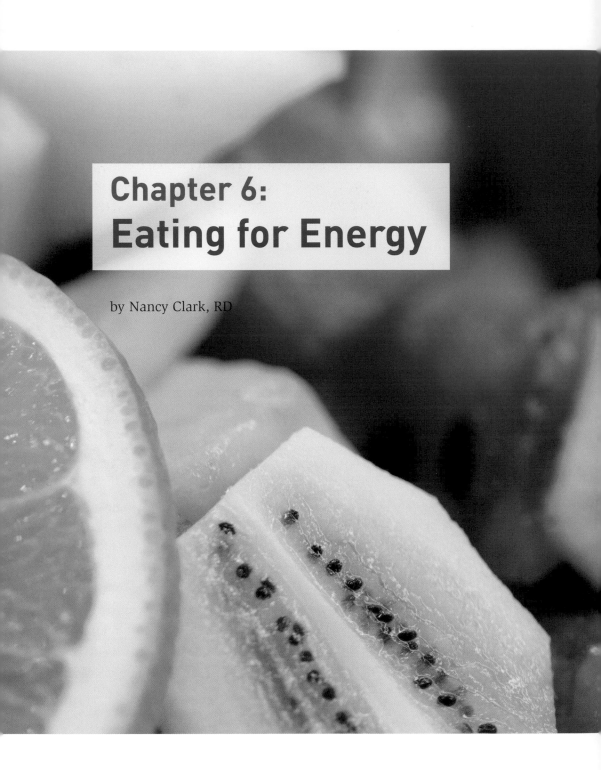

Chapter 6:
Eating for Energy

by Nancy Clark, RD

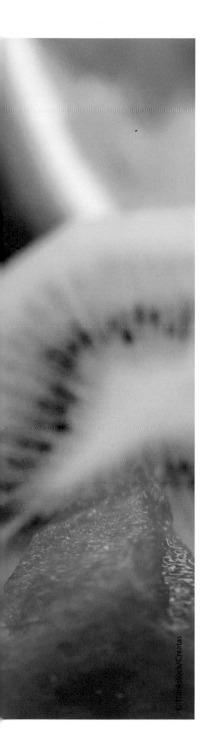

©Thinkstock/Creatas

Carbohydrates for Your Sports Diet

By eating grains, fruits, and vegetables as the foundation of each meal, you'll consume about 55 to 65% of your calories from carbohydrates. This is exactly what you need for a high-energy sports diet. These carbohydrates are stored in muscles in the form of glycogen, the energy you need to train hard day after day, and to compete well on race day.

Grain foods are a popular source of carbohydrates for most active people. But some marathoners believe they will get fat if they eat breads, cereals, and pastas at each meal. False! Carbohydrates are not fattening; excess calories are fattening. Your body needs carbs to fuel your muscles.

Fruits and vegetables are also great sources of carbohydrates. But eating the recommended 2 cups (500 g) of fruits and 2.5 cups (600 g) of vegetables is another story. As one marathoner sheepishly remarked, "I'm lucky if I eat that much in a week."

The trick is to eat large portions. Most runners can easily enjoy a banana (1 cup fruit, 240 g) and 8 oz (1 cup, 240 ml) of orange juice in the morning. That's the minimal fruit duty for the day! A big bowl of salad filled with colorful tomatoes, carrots, and peppers can account for the minimal recommended 2.5 cups of vegetables.

Balancing Your Diet

The trick to balancing the recommended servings of foods during your day is to plan to have at least three out of five food groups per meal, and one or two food groups per snack, such as:

	Breakfast	Lunch	Snack	Dinner	Snack
Grain	oatmeal	bread		spaghetti	popcorn
Fruit	raisins	banana	apple		juice
Vegetable			baby carrots	tomato sauce	
Dairy	(low-fat) milk		yogurt	cheese	parmesan
Protein	almonds	peanut butter	ground turkey		

If your goal is to be a strong runner in your golden years, today you want to start choosing meals abundant with fruits, vegetables, and whole-grain foods.

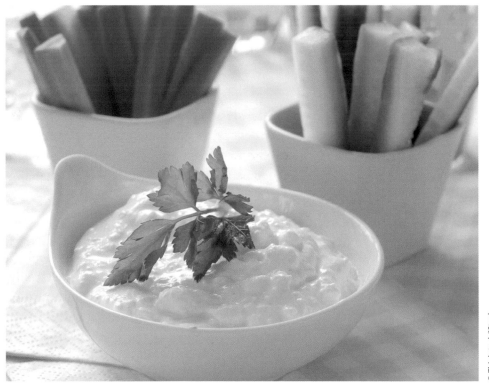

© Thinkstock/iStock

Fruits: Recommended Daily Intake—2 to 3 cups (500 - 700 g)

Each of these counts as 1 cup:

Orange juice 8 oz (240 ml)

Apple 1 small (100 g)

Banana 1 small (100 g)

Canned fruit 1 cup (240 g)

Dried fruit 1/2 cup (80 g)

Vegetables: Recommended Daily Intake—2.5 to 3+ cups (600- 700+ g)

Each of these counts as 1 cup:

Broccoli 1 medium stalk (200 g)

Spinach 2 cups (60 g)

Salad bar 1 average bowl (100 g)

Spaghetti sauce 1 cup (250 g)

Fruits and vegetables are truly nature's vitamin pills, chock full of vitamin C (to help with healing), beta-carotene (to protect against cancer), fiber (to aid with regular bowel movements), and numerous other vitamins and minerals.

Pasta

Every runner regardless of language understands the word pasta. Pasta parties are universally enjoyed around the world. Pasta is popular not only pre-marathon, but also as a standard part of the training diet. Even marathoners who claim they can't cook manage to boil pasta in one shape or another. Some choose to eat pasta at least five nights of the week thinking it is a kind of super food. Wrong.

Granted, pasta is carbohydrate-rich, quick and easy to cook, heart-healthy, economical, fun to eat, and enjoyed by just about every member of the family. But in terms of vitamins, minerals, and protein, plain pasta is a lackluster food.

Here's some information to help you to place pasta in perspective.

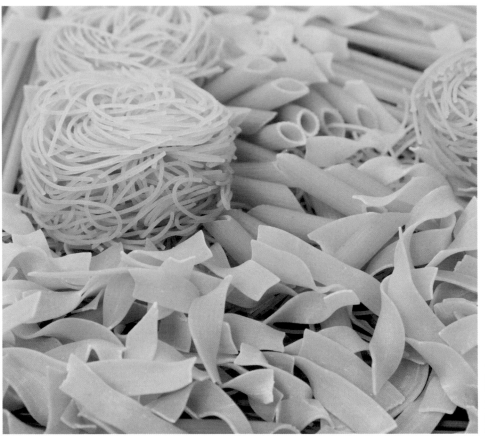

© Thinkstock/iStock

Nutritional value: Pasta is an excellent source of carbohydrates for muscle fuel and is the equivalent of "gas" for your engine. But plain pasta is a marginal source of vitamins and minerals, the "spark plugs" you need for top performance.

Pasta is simply made from refined white flour—the same stuff you get in "wonder breads"—with a few vitamins added to replace those lost during processing. Whole-wheat pastas offer a little nutritional boost, but wheat and other grains, in general, are better respected for their carbohydrate-value than their vitamins and minerals. Spinach and tomato pastas also are overrated since they contain relatively little spinach or tomato in comparison to having a serving of that vegetable along with the meal.

Pasta's nutritional value comes from the sauces:
- tomato sauce rich in vitamins A and C and potassium
- pesto-type sauces rich in vitamins A and C and potassium
- clam sauce rich in protein, zinc, and iron.

Be cautious with pasta smothered with butter, cream, or greasy meat sauces. Creamy, cheesy pastas can be artery-clogging nutritional nightmares.

Pasta and protein: Pasta is popular not only for carbohydrates but also for being a vegetarian alternative to meat-based meals. However, many marathoners live on too much pasta and neglect their protein needs. For example, Joe, an aspiring Olympian, thought his high-carbohydrate, low-fat diet of pasta and tomato sauce seven nights per week was top notch. He came to me wondering why he felt chronically tired and was not improving despite hard training.

The answer was simple. His limited diet was deficient in not only protein but also iron and zinc. Once he started to supplement the pasta with a variety of proteins, he started to feel better, run better, and recover better. He added to his tomato sauce a variety of protein-rich choices:
- extra-lean ground beef or turkey
- grated low-fat mozzarella cheese
- tofu
- canned, drained kidney beans
- canned tuna
- minced clams
- low-fat cottage cheese

Or, instead of adding protein to the sauce, he drank two glasses of low-fat milk with the meal.

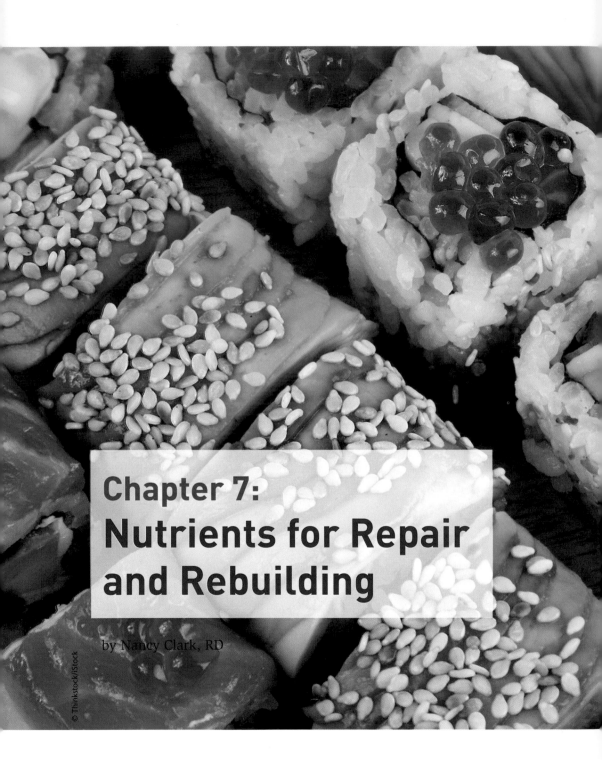

© Thinkstock/iStock

Chapter 7:
Nutrients for Repair and Rebuilding

by Nancy Clark, RD

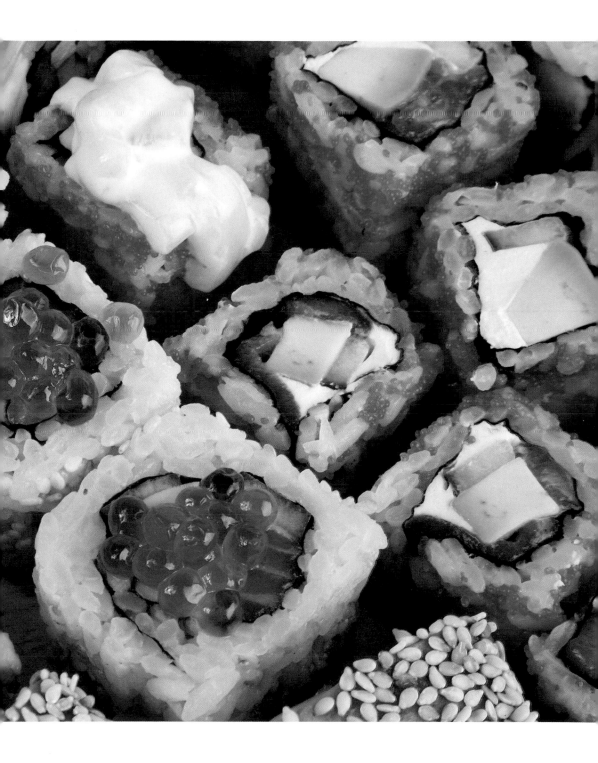

Protein for Your Sports Diet

Like carbohydrates, protein-rich foods are also an important part of your sports diet. You should eat a protein-rich food at each meal. Runners tend to either over- or underconsume protein, depending on their health consciousness and lifestyle.

Whereas some marathoners frequently choose pepperoni pizza, fast food burgers, and other meals filled with saturated fats, other runners bypass these foods in their efforts to eat a low-fat or vegetarian diet—but they neglect to replace beef with beans.

Recommended Daily Protein Intake: 5 to 7 oz (or ounce-equivalents; 140 to 200 g)

Runner's Protein-Rich Foods Portions (in Ounce or Ounce-Equivalents)
Tuna 6-oz (170 g) can drained (3-4 ounce-equivalents)
Chicken 6-oz breast (6)
Peanut butter 2-4 tablespoons (1-2)
Kidney beans 1 cup (4)

To meet your protein requirement for the day, you should consume a protein-rich food at each meal. Low-fat dairy foods such as milk, yogurt, and cheese (or other calcium-rich foods, such as calcium-fortified soy milk) offer a good way to boost your intake of high-quality protein as well as calcium. Calcium is important not only for growing teens and women who want to optimize bone density, but also men who want to have strong bones past the age of 70. For only 300 calories, all runners can easily contribute toward their protein intake plus achieve the recommended two to three servings of calcium-rich foods per day by consuming:

- 8 oz (240 ml) of milk or soy milk on breakfast cereal
- 8 oz (240 ml) of yogurt with lunch
- a (decaf) latte made with low-fat milk for an afternoon energizer

When choosing dairy foods, note that fat-free and low-fat products are preferable for heart health and calorie control, but you need not suffer with skim milk if you really don't like it. You can always cut back on fat in other parts of your diet. For example, Margie, a first-time marathoner, opted for cereal with reduced-fat (2%) milk (5 g of fat per cup), but saved on fat elsewhere in her diet by choosing low-fat cheese and mustard instead of mayonnaise on her sandwich.

Runners who prefer a dairy-free diet or are lactose intolerant should take special care to eat adequate amounts of non-dairy calcium sources or lactose-free milk.

Basic Shopping List

Keep this on our refrigerator and be sure to notice when an item gets low and needs to be replaced.

Cupboard: oatmeal, whole-grain cereals, pasta, spaghetti sauce, brown rice, whole-grain crackers, baked corn chips, kidney beans, baked beans, refried beans, chickpeas, tuna, canned salmon, peanut butter, soups (mushroom for making casseroles, lentil, minestrone, hearty bean), baking potatoes, V-8 and other vegetable juices

Refrigerator: low-fat cheddar, mozzarella and cottage cheese, low-fat milk or soymilk, (Greek) yogurt, Parmesan cheese, eggs, tofu, tortillas, baby carrots, lettuce, tomatoes, oranges, bananas (when refrigerated, the banana peel turns black but the fruit itself is fine and lasts longer), fresh fruit in season

Freezer: whole-grain bagels, pita, English muffins and bread, orange juice concentrate, strawberries, blueberries, broccoli, spinach, winter squash, ground turkey, extra-lean hamburger, chicken (pieces frozen individually in baggies)

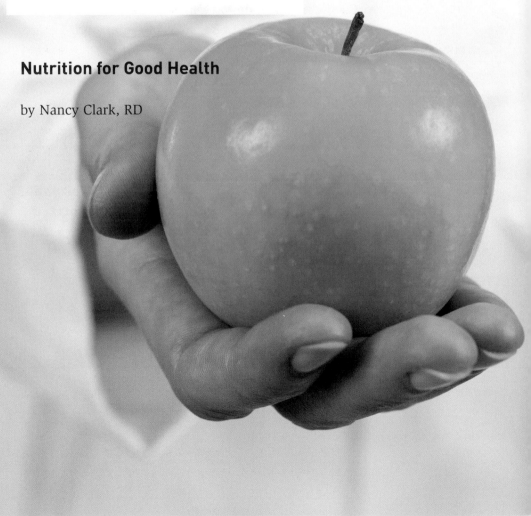

Chapter 8:
Healthy Eating Guidelines

Nutrition for Good Health

by Nancy Clark, RD

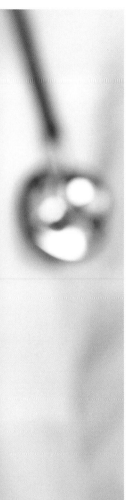

© Thinkstock/iStock

By following these dietary recommendations, you can substantially reduce your risk of developing heart disease and other diseases of aging.

- Balance calorie intake and physical activity to achieve and maintain a healthy bodyweight.
- Consume a diet rich in vegetables and fruits.
- Choose whole-grain, high-fiber foods.
- Consume fish, especially oily fish, at least twice a week.
- Limit your intake of saturated fat to < 7% of energy, trans fat to < 1% of energy, and cholesterol to < 300 mg per day
  - by choosing lean meats and vegetable alternatives
  - by selecting fat-free (skim), 1%-fat, and low-fat dairy products—minimizing intake of partially hydrogenated fats.
- Minimize your intake of beverages and foods with added sugars.
- Choose and prepare foods with little or no salt.
- If you consume alcohol, do so in moderation.
- When you eat food that is prepared outside of the home, follow these dietary recommendations.
- When selecting and preparing meat, poultry, dry beans, and milk or milk products, make choices that are lean, low-fat, or fat-free.
- Limit your intake of saturated and trans fats and choose healthier oils such as olive and canola oils, nuts and nut butters, and oily fish such as salmon.

Source: Diet and Lifestyle Recommendation Revision 2006: A Scientific Statement From the American Heart Association Nutrition Committee. A. Lichtenstein et all. Circulation 2006; 114:82-96.

Eat More Veggies!

If you struggle to consume the recommended two to three servings of vegetables per day, the following tips may help you enhance your vegetable intake—and your health.

- Eat more of the best vegetables, less of the rest. In general, dark green, deep yellow, orange, and red vegetables have far more nutrients than pale ones. Hence, if you dislike pale zucchini, summer squash, and cucumbers, don't work hard to acquire a taste for them. Instead, put your efforts into having more broccoli, spinach, and winter squash—the richly colored, more nutrient-dense choices.
- Eat colorful salads filled with tomatoes, green peppers, carrots, spinach, and dark lettuces. Pale salads with white lettuce, cucumbers, onions, celery, and other pale veggies offer little more than crunch. When smothered with dressing, this crunch becomes highly caloric. Alternatives to a pale restaurant salad include tomato juice, vegetable soup, a steamed veggie or, when you get home, a handful of raw baby carrots for a bedtime snack.
- Fortify spaghetti sauce with a (frozen) chopped broccoli or green peppers. Steam or microwave the veggies before you add them to the tomato sauce.

Sweets and Treats

Some marathoners eat far too many sweets and treats, even though they know they should be eating a wholesome diet based on grains, fruits, and vegetables. If you have a sweet tooth, you may be able correct this imbalance by eating larger portions of wholesome foods before you get too hungry. Marathoners who get too hungry tend to choose sugary, fatty foods (such as apple pie, instead of apples). A simple solution to sweet cravings is to prevent hunger by eating more wholesome food at meals.

Take Note: You need not eat a "perfect diet" (no fats, no sugar) to have a good diet. Nothing is nutritionally wrong with having a cookie for dessert after having eaten a sandwich, milk, and fruit for lunch. But a lot is wrong with skipping the sandwich and then eating cookies for lunch. That's when nutrition and performance problems arise.

The key to balancing fats and sugars appropriately in your diet is to abide by the following guidelines:

- 10% of your calories can come from refined sugar, if desired (about 200–300 calories from sugar per day for most runners)
- 25% of your calories can appropriately come from fat (about 450–750 calories from fat per day, or roughly 50–85 grams of fat per day)

Hence, moderate amounts of chips, cookies, and ice cream can fit into an overall healthful food plan.

- Choose fast foods with the most veggies:
  - pizza with peppers, mushrooms, and extra tomato sauce
  - Chinese entrees stir-fried with vegetables
- lunchtime V-8 juice instead of diet soda
- Even over-cooked vegetables are better than no vegetables. If your only option is over- cooked veggies from the cafeteria, eat them. While cooking does destroy some of the vegetable's nutrients, it does not destroy all of them. Any vegetable is better than no vegetable!
- Keep frozen vegetables stocked in your freezer, ready and waiting. They are quick and easy to prepare, won't spoil quickly, and have more nutrients than "fresh" vegetables that have been in the market and then your refrigerator for a few days. Because cooking (more than freezing) reduces a vegetable's nutritional content:
  - quickly cook vegetables only until tender crisp and use the cooking water as a broth
  - microwave vegetables in a covered dish
  - stir-fry them with a little olive oil.
- When all else fails, eat fruit to help compensate for lack of vegetables. The best alternatives include bananas, oranges, grapefruit, melon, berries, and kiwi. These choices are rich in many of the same nutrients found in vegetables.

Need Some Help Shaping Up Your Diet?

If you want personalized dietary advice, I recommend that you seek professional advice from a registered dietitian (RD) who specializes in sports nutrition and, ideally, is board certified as a specialist in sports dietetics (CSSD). To find a sports dietitian in your area, use the referral networks on the Academy of Nutrition and Dietetics website (www.eatright.org) or the website of ADA's practice group of sports dietitians (www.SCANdpg.org). Or try googling "sports nutritionist" or "sports dietitian" in your city. You'll be glad you did! This personal nutrition coach can help you enjoy miles of smiles and years of good health.

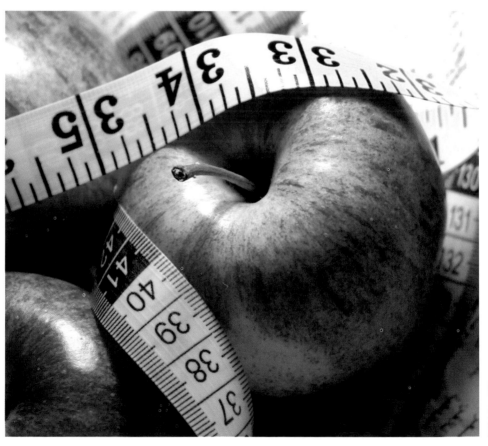

© Thinkstock/Hemera

Calcium Equivalents

The recommended daily calcium intake is:

Age group   Calcium (mg)
Teens 9-18 years   1,300
Adults 19-50 years   1,000
Adults 51 + years   1,200
Source: Dietary Reference Intakes, National Academy of Science, 1997

The following foods all provide about 300 mg of calcium. Three choices per day, or one at each meal, will contribute to meeting your calcium needs.

Calcium-Rich Dairy Foods and Amounts
- milk, whole or skim 1 cup (240 ml)
- yogurt, 1 cup (230 g)
- cheese, 1 1/2 oz (45 g)
- cottage cheese, 2 cups (450 g)
- frozen yogurt, 1 1/2 cups (150 g)

Proteins
- soy milk,* 1 cup (240 ml)
- tofu, 8 oz (1/2 cake; 250 g)
- salmon, canned with bones 5 oz (140 g)
- sardines, canned with bones 3 oz (85 g)
- almonds, 4 oz (110 g)

Vegetables
- Broccoli, cooked 3 cups (550 g)
- Collard or turnip greens, cooked 1 cup (150 g)
- Kale or mustard greens, cooked 1 1/2 cups (220 g)

Check label to be sure the food has added protein.

Calcium-fortified foods*
- Orange juice, 8 oz
- Rice milk, 8 oz
- Almond milk, 8 oz

*Check label to be sure the food has added calcium.

Vegetables 101: Basic Cooking Tips

Vegetables are nutrient-rich, but cooking can destroy some of their nutritional value. To get the most nutrients from your vegetables, handle them properly so they have minimal exposure to air, heat, water, and light—the four elements that reduce their nutritional value.

- To reduce exposure to air: Store fresh vegetables in plastic containers. Cook covered.
- To reduce exposure to heat: Store fresh vegetables in the refrigerator; minimize cooking time to enhance the flavor and nutritional value.
- To reduce exposure to water: Cook in minimal water, stir-fry, or microwave.
- To reduce exposure to light: Store in a dark place (inside the fridge!); cook in a covered pan.

Basic Steamed Vegetables
1. Wash vegetables thoroughly; prepare and cut into pieces keeping the skin or peel, if appropriate.
2. Put 1/2-inch (1 cm) water in the bottom of a pan that has a tight cover.
3. Bring the water to a boil. Add the vegetables. Or, put the vegetables in a steamer basket and put this in the saucepan with 1 inch (2 cm) of water.
4. Cover the pan tightly and cook over medium heat until the vegetables are tender crisp, about 3 minutes for spinach, 10 minutes for broccoli, and 15 minutes for sliced carrots.
5. Drain the vegetables, reserving the cooking water for soup or sauces, or simply drink it as a broth.

Summary

Nutrition for running is all about fueling with a purpose so you can then enjoy the benefits of high energy and good health. Your food goals are to eat at least three kinds of wholesome foods at each meal, at least two kinds of wholesome foods for each snack; evenly-sized meals about every four hours throughout the day (as opposed to "crescendo eating" with a small breakfast and a large meal at the end of the day); at least 90% of the calories from quality foods and, if desired, the remaining 10% from sweets and treats.

You need not eat a "perfect diet" to have a good diet, but you do want to choose more of the best foods (wholesome grains, fruits, vegetables, low-fat dairy, lean meats, beans, and plant-sources of protein) and less of the rest.

If you wish to add some seasonings before or after cooking, here are some nice combinations:
- Basil: green beans, tomatoes, zucchini
- Oregano: zucchini, mushrooms, tomatoes, onions
- Dill: green beans, carrots, peas, potatoes
- Cinnamon: spinach, winter squash, sweet potatoes
- Marjoram: celery, greens
- Nutmeg: corn, cauliflower, green beans
- Thyme: artichokes, mushrooms, peas, carrots
- Parsley: sprinkled on any vegetable

Basic Microwaved Vegetables

Microwave cookery is perfect for vegetables because microwaves cook the veggies quickly and without water, thereby retaining a greater percentage of the nutrients than with conventional methods.

1. Wash the vegetables and cut them into bite-size pieces. Put them in a microwavable container with a cover.
2. Microwave until tender crisp; stir halfway through cooking, so they cook evenly. The amount of time will vary according to your particular microwave oven and the amount of vegetable you are cooking. Start off with three minutes for a single serving; larger servings take longer. The

vegetables will continue cooking after you remove them from the oven, so plan that into your cooking time.

Basic Stir-Fried Vegetables

Vegetables stir-fried until tender crisp are very flavorful, colorful, and nutritious, but they do have more calories than if steamed. If weight is an issue, be sure to add only a minimal amount of oil (olive, canola, sesame) to the cooking pan.

Some popular stir-fry combinations include:
- Carrots, broccoli, and mushrooms
- Onions, green peppers, zucchini, and tomatoes
- Chinese cabbage, bok choy, and water chestnuts

1. Wash, drain well (to prevent the water from spattering when the vegetables are added to the hot cooking oil), and cut the vegetables of your choice into bite-sized pieces or 1/8-inch slices. Whenever possible, slice vegetables diagonally to increase the surface area; this allows for faster cooking. Try to make the pieces uniform so they will cook evenly.
2. Heat the skillet over high heat. Add 1 to 3 teaspoons of oil, just enough to coat the bottom of the pan. Optional: Add a slice of ginger root or some minced garlic, stir-frying for 1 minute to add flavor.
3. Add the vegetables that take longest to cook (carrots, cauliflower, broccoli); a few minutes later add the remaining ones (mushrooms, bean sprouts, cabbage, spinach). Constantly lift and turn the vegetables to coat them with oil.
4. Add a little bit of water (1/4-1/2 cup), then cover and steam the vegetables for 2 to 5 minutes. Adjust the heat to prevent scorching.
5. Don't overcrowd the pan. Cook small batches at a time.
6. Optional add-ins: soy sauce, stir-fried beef, chicken, tofu, rice, or noodles.
7. To thicken the juices, stir in a mixture of 2 teaspoons cornstarch diluted into 1 tablespoon water. Add more water or broth if this makes the sauce too thick.

Optional: Garnish with toasted sesame seeds, mandarin orange sections, or pineapple chunks.

Basic Baked Vegetables

If you are baking chicken, potatoes, or a casserole, you might as well make good use of the oven and bake the vegetables, too.

Some popular suggestions include:
- Eggplant halves sprinkled with garlic powder
- Zucchini with onions and oregano
- Carrots with ginger
- Sliced sweet potato with apple

1. Put the vegetables (seasoned as desired) in a covered baking dish with a small amount of water, or wrap them in foil.
2. Bake at 350°F (175°C) for 20 to 30 minutes (depending on the size of the chunks) until tender crisp. Caution: With foil-wrapped vegetables, be careful when opening the foil. The escaping steam might burn you.

Adapted from: *Nancy Clark's Sports Nutrition Guidebook,* Fourth Edition (Human Kinetics, 2008).

Vitamins and Minerals

More than half of Americans take dietary supplements in the belief that they will make them feel better, give them greater energy, improve their health, and prevent and treat disease. Users spend more than $23 billion a year on dietary supplements; the vitamin industry is a booming business.

Vitamins are essential substances that your body can't make. They perform important jobs in your body, including helping to convert food into energy. (Vitamins do not provide energy, however; carbohydrates do.) Although a supplement is certainly a quick and easy safety net for hit-or-miss eating, I highly recommend that you first make the effort to "eat" your vitamins via natural foods. As a hungry runner who requires more calories than the average person, you can easily consume large doses of vitamins in, let's say, a taller glass of orange juice or bigger pile of steamed broccoli.

Because food consumption surveys suggest that many people fail to eat a well-balanced variety of wholesome foods, some runners and walkers may indeed suffer from marginal nutritional deficiencies, particularly those who:
- restrict calories,
- eat a repetitive diet of rice cakes and apples,
- skimp on fruits, vegetables, and dairy foods, and
- over-indulge in fats and sweets.

Even marathoners who believe they eat well sometimes miss the mark. For example, one woman who took pride in her high-carbohydrate, low-fat diet (primarily bagels, bananas, pasta, and pretzels) ate too many carbohydrates at the exclusion of other foods (such as meats and dairy). She had a diet deficient in calcium, iron, zinc, and protein.

As a result of American's unbalanced food choices, should the general public be encouraged to take a supplement to compensate for poor eating habits? Not necessarily. Despite the rising popularity of supplements, many health organizations, including the American Heart Association and the National Institutes of Health, recommend food, not pills, for optimal nutrition. That's because food contains far more than just vitamins. It contains phytochemicals, fiber, and other health-protective substances that are not in pills. Hence, the key to good health is to learn how to eat well despite a hectic lifestyle.

Let's take a look at some of what is and what is not known about nutritional supplements, and hopefully you'll see why spending more money on broccoli and orange juice rather than on pills and potions is the wiser bet. Whole foods offer protein, carbohydrates, fiber, and phytochemicals—far more than just vitamins and minerals.

Vitamins were originally studied to determine the minimal amount of a nutrient required to prevent deficiency diseases such as beriberi and scurvy. The recommended dietary allowances were developed to guide people towards an appropriate intake; they include a large safety margin. For example, in the US, the Dietary Reference Intake (DRI) for vitamin C is 75 to 90 mg (women, men); this is four times the minimal amount needed to prevent the deficiency disease scurvy. The question remains unanswered: What is the optimal level of vitamins, not just to prevent deficiency, but also to enhance health?

No amount of any supplement will compensate for a high-fat, hit-or-miss diet and stress-filled lifestyle.

But supplements are indeed appropriate for certain populations, including:
- folic acid for pregnant women and women who might become pregnant (expectedly or unexpectedly), to prevent certain birth defects,
- iron for vegetarians and women with heavy menstrual periods,
- zinc and antioxidants for nonsmokers with macular degeneration (an eye),
- vitamin D and calcium for postmenopausal women for strong bones,
- vitamin D for people who live in northern latitudes.

To date, no studies have documented a physiological need for mega-doses of vitamins, even for marathoners and other athletes. Most athletes can consume more than enough vitamins through their daily food intake.

Runners who eat vitamin-enriched energy bars and breakfast cereals, as well as other enriched grain foods, commonly consume far more vitamins than they realize.

Note: runners who eat primarily "all natural foods" from the whole foods stores miss out on the benefit of enriched foods. ("All natural foods" have no added vitamins or minerals, like iron.) That's one reason why the government acknowledges that some of our grains can appropriately come from enriched foods.

Food Offers More Than Vitamins

Whole foods such as fruits and vegetables offer hundreds, perhaps thousands, of substances called phytochemicals that protect our health. These include:
- *protease inhibitors* in soybeans that may slow tumor growth
- *isoflavones* in dried beans that may reduce the risk of breast or ovarian cancer
- *isothiocyanates* in broccoli that may help block carcinogens from damaging a cell's DNA

These phytochemicals may explain why the cruciferous vegetables such as broccoli, cabbage, and cauliflower are thought to be protective against cancer, and onions and garlic are thought to be protective against heart disease. Deeply colored, antioxidant-rich fruits such as tart cherries, blueberries, grape juice, and pomegranate juice can enhance your health and recovery from exercise. Yet, taking high doses of antioxidant supplements such as vitamins C and E may create an imbalance that has a negative effect on your immune system.

While not a vitamin, omega-3 fish oil is another nutrient found in food that is powerfully health protective. The American Heart Association recommends that healthy people eat 12 oz (two to three servings) of preferably oily fish, such as salmon and tuna, each week to provide the omega-3 fats that protect against heart disease. For non-fish eaters, flaxseed, walnuts, and canola oil can be plant-based alternatives. Take heed: Even fit marathoners are not immune from heart disease!

As you decide your nutritional fate, know that a diet based on a variety of wholesome foods is your best source of good nutrition. If you choose to take a supplement for its potential health-protective effects, be sure to do so in *addition to eating well*. Because researchers have yet to unravel the whole vitamin/health mystery, stay tuned and be sure to take care of your whole health. The phytochemicals, omega-3 fats, and other unknown substances found in whole foods, but not in pills, tend to emerge as the winner.

Am I sick? Am I tired? Do I Need Vitamins?

Exercise energizes many people, enhancing their productivity as well as relieving their stress. But some runners complain of chronic fatigue. They feel run down, dragged out, and overwhelmingly exhausted. If this sounds familiar, you may wonder if you are sick, overtired, or if something is wrong with your diet. You may wonder if taking vitamins would solve the problem.

Perhaps you can relate to Peter, a 39-year-old marathon runner, lawyer, and solo chef who bemoaned, "I just don't take the time to eat right. My diet is awful. I rarely eat fruits or vegetables, to say nothing of a real meal. I think that poor nutrition is catching up with me. What vitamins should I take?"

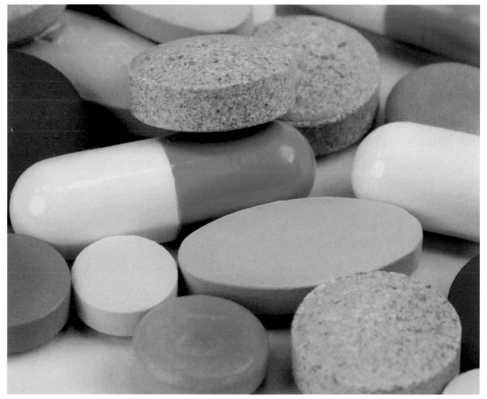

© Thinkstock/iStock

Peter lived alone, hated to cook for just himself, tended to survive on fast (and fatty) foods. He rarely ate breakfast, barely ate lunch, but always collapsed after a long day with a generous feast of a large deli sandwich, Chinese take-out, or pizza. He struggled to wake up in the morning, to stay awake during afternoon meetings, and to grind through his daily 10 mile run.

I evaluated Peter's diet, calculated that he required about 3,000 calories per day (700 to 800 calories per meal—breakfast, lunch #1, lunch #2, dinner), and suggested a few simple food changes that could result in higher energy, greater stamina, and better running. Trying to find some solutions to Peter's fatigue, I explored the following questions. Perhaps the answers will offer solutions for your energy problems.

- **Are you tired due to low blood sugar?** Peter skipped not only breakfast but also often missed lunch because he "didn't have time." He would doze off in the afternoon because he had low blood sugar. With zero calories to feed his brain, he ended up feeling sleepy.

The solution was to choose to make time to eat. Just as he chose to sleep later in the morning, he could choose to stock trail mix (granola, nuts, and raisins) at the office, so he could munch on that for his morning fuel. He could also choose to stop working for 5 or 10 minutes to eat lunch.

- **Is your diet too low in carbohydrates?** Peter's fast-but-fatty food choices filled his stomach but left his muscles poorly fueled with inadequate glycogen to support his training program. Higher carbohydrate snacks and meals would not only fuel his muscles but also help maintain a normal blood sugar level, thereby providing energy for mental work as well as physical exercise.

- **Are you iron-deficient and anemic?** Peter ate little red meat and consequently little iron, an important mineral in red blood cells that helps carry oxygen to exercising muscles. Iron-deficiency anemia can

© Thinkstock/Creatas

result in needless fatigue during exercise. I taught Peter how to boost his dietary iron intake, with or without meat. I also recommended he talk to his doctor about getting his blood tested (hemoglobin, hematocrit, ferritin, serum iron, and total iron-binding capacity) to rule out the question of anemia.

- **Are you getting enough sleep?** Peter's complaint about being chronically tired was justified because he was tired both mentally (from his intense job) and physically (from his strenuous training) tired. He worked from 8 a.m. to 8 p.m. By the time he got home, ran, ate dinner, and unwound, midnight had rolled around. The wake-up bell at 6:30 a.m. came all too soon—especially since Peter often had trouble falling asleep due to having eaten such a large dinner.

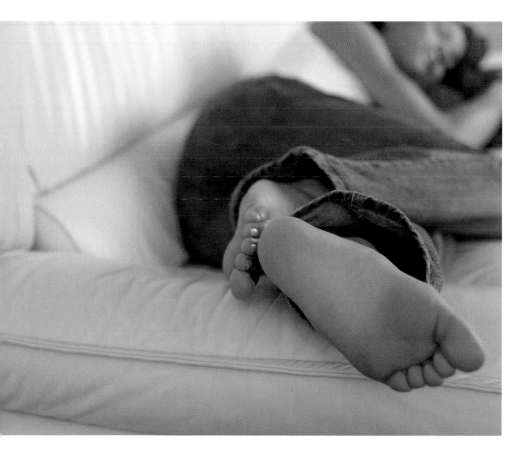

I recommended that Peter try to get more sleep by eating lighter dinners (soup and sandwich, or even cereal), having bigger breakfasts, and scheduling his main meal at noon (low-fat Chinese meals, vegetable soup and hearty sandwich, or pasta).

By trading in 1,200 of his evening calories for 600 more calories at breakfast and 600 more calories at lunch, he could determine if less food in his stomach before bed would result in better sleep.

- **Are you overtraining?** Although Peter took pride in the fact that he hadn't missed a day of running in seven years, he felt discouraged he wasn't improving despite harder training. I questioned whether he was a "compulsive runner" who punished his body or a "serious athlete" who trained wisely and took rest days. One or two rest days or easy days per week are an essential part of a training program; they allow the muscles to heal and to replenish their depleted glycogen stores.

- **Are you stressed or depressed?** Peter not only had a stressful job, he was also dealing with the stress and depression associated with family problems, to say nothing of the challenges of training for a marathon. Since he was feeling a bit helpless with this situation, I encouraged him to successfully control at least one aspect of his life—his diet. Simple dietary improvements would help him feel better not only physically but also mentally. This would be very energizing in itself.

If you answered "yes" to many of the questions I asked Peter, you may be able to resolve your fatigue with better eating, sleeping, and training habits—not with vitamin pills. Experiment with the simple food suggestions in this book. Before long you may transform your current low-energy patterns into a food plan for success! Eating well is not as hard as you may think.

Summary

Your best bet for fighting fatigue is to be responsible with your food choices and nourish your body with the right balance of wholesome foods. Make the effort to eat a variety of foods and fluids from the different food groups every day. Eating marathoner's portions, you will consume not only the amounts of the vitamins and minerals you need, you will also be giving your body the calories it needs to prevent fatigue.

If you are tempted to take supplements for health insurance, do so only if you simultaneously choose to eat a healthful diet. Remember, no amount of supplements will compensate for an inadequate diet—but you will always win with good nutrition. Eat wisely, eat well!

For more information

Confusion abounds regarding dietary supplements, their safety, and their potential health benefits. Here are some websites that offer abundant information about vitamins and health. You might need to do a search on "vitamins" or "fish oil" to find your topic of interest within each website:
The American Heart Association: www.americanheart.org
FDA's Center for Food Safety and Applied Nutrition www.cfsan.fda.gov
National Library of Medicine: www.nlm.nih.gov/medlineplus
The World's Healthiest Foods: www.whfoods.org

Chapter 9:
Breakfast—
The Meal of
Champions

by Nancy Clark, RD

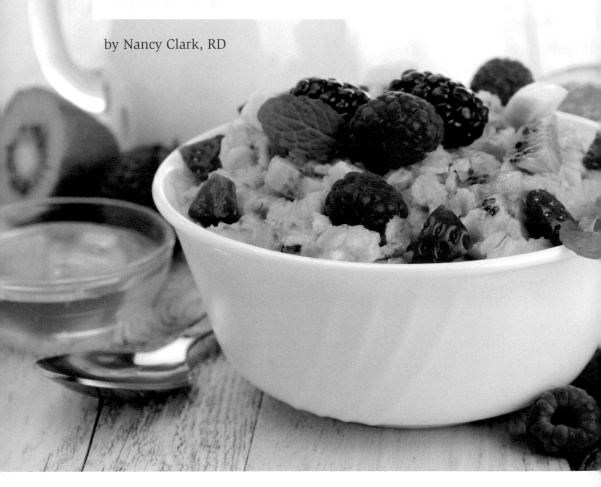

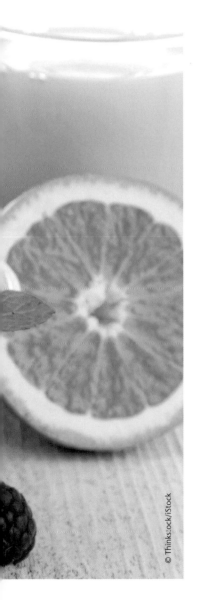

© Thinkstock/iStock

Eating breakfast means you have to find the desire to do so. You'll want to eat breakfast as you observe that the benefits of eating a proper breakfast far outweigh the costs. Breakfast eaters tend to:

- **eat a more nutrient-dense and overall better diet the rest of the day (a wholesome breakfast can reduce the urge for junk food at night),**

- **have lower blood cholesterol levels,**

- **enjoy success with weight control (in one survey, 88% of dieters who lost weight and kept it off became religious breakfast eaters; only 4% rarely ate breakfast) (Wyatt, 2002),**

- **are mentally alert and more productive (just like school kids who eat breakfast),**

- **have more energy to enjoy exercise either in the morning or later that day.**

As an athlete, you should eat even-sized meals about every four hours, starting with breakfast within three hours of waking. From petite female runners on a 2,000-calorie per day weight reduction diet, to tall men who devour 3,600 calories per day, marathoners require a hefty 500 to 900 calories for their morning fuel. (See chapter 16 for information on how to calculate your calorie needs for breakfast and the entire day.)

Morning runners commonly split their breakfast into a pre-run snack, such as a banana, followed by the recovery meal, such as a bagel with peanut butter on their way to the office. By spending one-fourth of your calories in the morning, you have adequate energy to start your busy day, to say nothing of abating hunger and the 10:00 a.m. hungry horrors.

Despite my clear message about breakfast being the most important meal of the day, I have to coax my clients to experiment with eating (more) breakfast. Far too many runners under-eat in the morning. Some fear if they eat more at breakfast, they'll get fat. Or if they eat breakfast, they'll feel more hungry than if they abstain. Let's take a look at some standard breakfast excuses—and solutions.

I don't have time: Lack of priority is the real problem, not lack of time. If you can make time to train, you can make time to fuel for your training. Even if you choose to sleep to the last minute before dragging yourself out of bed, you can still choose to eat breakfast on the way to work. Breakfast need not be an elaborate occasion.

You can quickly prepare a simple breakfast to eat on the run:
- a baggie filled with raisins, almonds, and granola.
- a wrap rolled with a slice or two of low-fat cheese.
- a peanut butter and honey sandwich on wholesome bread.
- a glass of milk, then a banana while walking to the bus or train.
- a travel mug filled with a fruit smoothie or protein shake (there will always be coffee at the office).
- an energy bar and some grapes during the morning commute.

The key to breakfast on the run is to plan ahead. Prepare your breakfast the night before so that you can simply grab it and go during the morning rush. For example, on the weekends, you might want to make banana bread or buy a dozen bagels. Pre-slice the bread or the bagels, wrap the desired portion in individual plastic bags, and put them in the freezer. Take one out of the freezer at night so breakfast will be ready and waiting in the morning.

Breakfast interferes with my training schedule: If you are an early morning runner or walker (5:00–7:00 a.m.), you will likely exercise better and avoid an energy crash if you eat part of your breakfast before you exercise (assuming your stomach can tolerate food, of course). Coffee with extra milk, a swig of juice, half a bagel, or a slice of toast are popular choices that can get your blood sugar on the upswing, contribute to greater stamina, and help you feel more awake. If you prefer to abstain, at least have a hefty bedtime snack the night before to help bolster your morning blood sugar.

Breakfast is equally important if you exercise at mid-day or in the afternoon. You need to fuel up in order to do a quality workout that afternoon.
Breakfast is essential if you are doing double workouts. Because your muscles are hungriest for carbohydrates within the first hour after hard exercise, a quick and easy recovery breakfast will set the stage for a strong second workout.

I sometimes hear runners express concern that eating breakfast interferes with their upcoming workout, that the food will sit heavily in the stomach or "talk back." This is unlikely. A low-fat meal at 7:00 to 8:00 a.m. (such as cereal and low-fat milk) should be well digested by noontime. Try it; you'll probably see a positive difference in your energy level.

I'm not hungry in the morning: If you have no morning appetite, the chances are you ate your breakfast calories the night before. Huge dinner? Ice cream? Too many cookies before bedtime? The solution to having no morning appetite is, obviously, to eat less at night so that you can start the day off hungry. If running first thing in the morning "kills your appetite" (due to the rise in body temperature), keep in mind that you will be hungry within a few hours when you have cooled down. Plan ahead, so when the hungry horrors hit, you will have healthful options ready and waiting. Otherwise, you'll be likely to grab whatever's easy, which may include doughnuts, pastries, and other high-fat foods.

I'm on a diet: Too many weight-conscious runners start their diet at breakfast. Bad idea. Breakfast skippers tend to gain weight and to be heavier than breakfast eaters. A satisfying breakfast prevents you from getting too hungry and overeating.

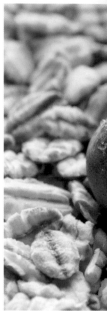

Your best bet for successful dieting is to eat during the day, burn off the calories, and then eat a lighter meal at night.

Breakfast makes me hungrier: Many runners complain that if they eat breakfast, they seem to get hungrier and eat more all day. This may result from thinking they have already "blown their diets" by eating breakfast, so they might as well keep overeating, then start dieting again the next day. Wrong.

Successful diets start at breakfast. If you feel hungry after breakfast you probably ate too little breakfast. For example, 100 calories of toast with jam is enough to whet your appetite but not to satisfy your calorie needs. Try budgeting about one-quarter of your calories for breakfast—500-600 calories for most 120-150 pound runners. This translates into two slices of toast with jam, a banana, low-fat yogurt, and juice; or yogurt and a bagel with peanut butter.

Note: If you overeat at breakfast, you can easily resolve the problem by eating less at lunch or dinner. You won't be as physically hungry for those meals and will be able to easily eat smaller portions.

The Breakfast of Champions

By now, I hope I've convinced you that breakfast is indeed the most important meal of the day for marathoners. What should you eat, you wonder? If you feel like cooking, enjoy hot oatmeal, French toast, or pancakes.

But if you are looking for a cook-free choice, I highly recommend cereal. Cereal is quick, convenient, and filled with the calcium, iron, carbohydrates, fiber, and other nutrients active people need. A bowl of bran cereal with fruit

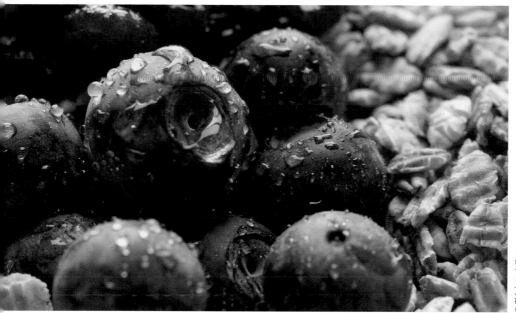

© Thinkstock/Fuse

and low-fat milk provides a well-balanced meal that includes three of the five food groups (grain, milk, and fruit) and sets the stage for an overall low-fat diet.

Cereal is versatile. You can eat it dry if you're on the run, or preferably with low-fat milk or yogurt for a calcium booster. You can mix brands and vary the flavor with different toppings:

- sliced banana
- blueberries (a handful of frozen ones taste great—especially if microwaved)
- raisins
- canned fruit
- cinnamon
- maple syrup
- vanilla yogurt

My personal favorite is to put a mix of cereals in my bowl, top it with fruit, heat it in the microwave oven for 30 to 60 seconds, and then add cold milk. It's like eating fruit cobbler!

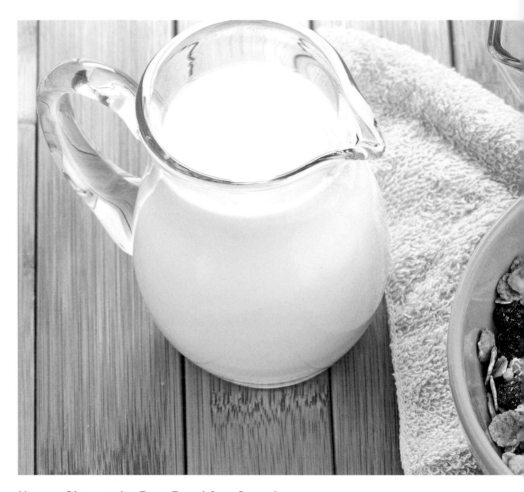

How to Choose the Best Breakfast Cereal

Needless to say, all cereals are not created equal. Some offer more nutritional value than others. Here are four tips to help you make the best choices.

1. Choose iron-enriched cereals with at least 25% of the daily value for iron to help prevent anemia.

Note, however, the iron in breakfast cereals is poorly absorbed compared to the iron in lean red meats. But you can enhance iron absorption by drinking a glass of orange juice or enjoying another source of vitamin C (such as grapefruit, cantaloupe, strawberries, or kiwi) along with the cereal. Any iron is better than no iron.

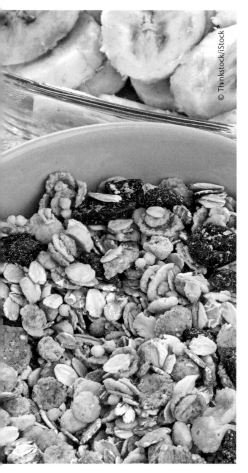

© Thinkstock/iStock

If you tend to eat "all-natural" types of cereals, such as granola and shredded wheat, be aware that these types have "no additives," hence no added iron. You might want to mix and match all-natural brands with iron enriched brands (or make the effort to eat iron-rich foods at other meals).

2. Choose fiber-rich bran cereals with more than 5 g of fiber per serving.
Fiber not only helps prevent constipation but also is a protective nutrient that may reduce your risk of colon cancer and heart disease. Bran cereals are the best sources of fiber, more so than even fruits and vegetables. Choose from All-Bran, 40% Bran Flakes, Raisin Bran, Bran Chex, Fiber One or any of the numerous cereals with "bran" or "fiber" in the name. You can also mix high- and low-fiber cereals (Rice Crispies + Fiber One; Special K + Raisin Bran) to boost their fiber value.

Note: If you have trouble with diarrhea when running, you may want to forgo bran cereals. The extra fiber may aggravate the situation.

3. Choose cereals with whole grains listed among the first ingredients.
Whole grains include whole wheat, brown rice, corn, and oats; these should be listed first in the ingredients. In my opinion, you should pay more attention to a cereal's grain content than its sugar or sodium (salt) content. Here's why:

- Sodium is a concern primarily for people with high blood pressure. Most runners have low blood pressure and are unlikely to suffer health consequences from choosing cereals with a little added salt. Plus, runners who sweat heavily lose sodium and need to replace it.

- Sugar is simply a carbohydrate that fuels your muscles. Yes, sugar calories are nutritionally empty calories. But when sugar is combined with milk, banana, and the cereal itself, the twenty empty calories in 5 g of added sugar are insignificant. Obviously, sugar-filled frosted flakes and kids' cereals with 15 g of sugar or more per serving are more like dessert than breakfast. Hence, try to limit your breakfast choices to cereals with fewer than 5 g of added sugar per serving. Enjoy the sugary ones for snacks or dessert, if desired, or mix a little with low-sugar cereals.

4. Choose primarily low-fat cereals with less than 2 g of fat per serving.
High-fat cereals such as some brands of granola and crunchy cookie-type cereals can add unexpected fat and calories to your sports diet. Select low-fat brands for the foundation of your breakfast, and then use only a sprinkling of the higher-fat treats, if desired, for a topping.

Mix 'n Match Cereals
When it comes to cereals, you may not find one that meets all of your standards for whole grain, high fiber, high iron, and low fat, but you can always mix-and-match to create a winning combination.

Brand Iron	(%DV)	Fiber (g)	Fat (g)
"Ideal cereal"	> 25%	> 5	< 2
Cheerios 1 cup (30g)	45%	3	2
Wheaties, 1 cup (30 g)	45%	3	1
Kashi Go Lean, 1 cup (52 g)	10%	10	1
Raisin Bran, Kellogg's, 1 cup (59 g)	25%	7	1.5
Fiber One, 1/2 cup (30 g)	25%	14	1
Quaker 100% Natural 1/2 cup (48 g)	6%	3	6
Oat Squares, Quaker 1 cup (60 g)	90%	5	2.5
Cap'n Crunch 3/4 cup (30 g)	25%	1	1.5

Nontraditional Breakfasts

Not everyone likes cereal for breakfast, nor do they want to cook eggs or pancakes. If you are stumped by what to eat for breakfast, choose a food that you enjoy. After all, you'll be more likely to eat breakfast if it tastes good. Remember that any food—even a cookie (preferably oatmeal raisin, rather than chocolate chip)—is better than nothing.

How about:
- leftover pizza
- leftover Chinese food
- mug of tomato soup
- potato zapped in the microwave while you take your shower
- tuna sandwich
- peanut butter and apple
- protein bar

Summary

What you eat in the morning provides fuel for a high-energy day and stronger workouts. Breakfast helps novice and experienced marathoners alike to make their way to the winners' circle! Even dieters can enjoy breakfast without the fear of "getting fat"—that is, breakfast helps curb evening appetite so that dieters can eat lighter at night.

If you generally skip breakfast, at least give breakfast a try during your marathon training. You'll soon learn why breakfast is the meal of champions!

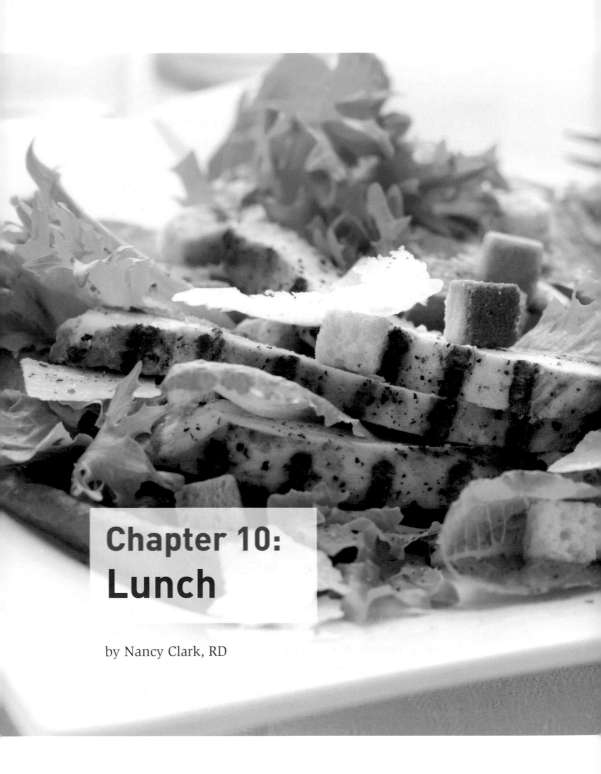

Chapter 10:
Lunch

by Nancy Clark, RD

Whereas breakfast is the most important meal of your training diet, lunch is the second most important meal. In fact, I encourage runners to eat TWO lunches! One lunch at 11:00 a.m., when you first start to get hungry, then a second lunch about 3:00 or 4:00 in the afternoon, when the munchies strike. If you train in the morning, these lunches refuel your muscles. If you train in the late afternoon, these lunches prepare you for a strong workout. And in either case, two lunches curb your appetite so you are not starving at the end of the day and have the energy to cook a nutritious dinner.

I invite you to experiment with this two-lunch concept. If you are like most of my clients, you'll find yourself looking forward to a second sandwich to boost your energy at the end of the day. Afraid that two lunches will be fattening? Fear not; a second lunch does not mean additional calories. You'll simply be trading your afternoon cookies and evening ice cream for a wholesome afternoon meal. No longer will you search for evening snacks; you won't be hungry for them.

What's for Lunch?

Runners commonly have three options for lunch: pack your own, pick up some fast food, or enjoy a hot meal from the cafeteria at work or school. You can eat healthfully in each of these scenarios; just remember to enjoy three kinds of wholesome food with each meal (bread + peanut butter + banana; pizza crust + tomato sauce + cheese; chicken + rice + vegetables) and at least 500 to 600 calories per meal (based on a 2,000 to 2,400 calorie food plan, the amount appropriate for marathoners who want to lose weight; non-dieters can target about 600 to 800 calories per meal).

© Thinkstock/iStock

Eating a hot meal in the middle of the day can make dinnertime easier for runners who train in the late afternoon, arrive home starved, and don't feel like cooking. By enjoying a nice meal at noon, you'll be content to have a simple supper, such as soup-and-sandwich.

Pack Your Own Lunches

Packing you own lunch is a good way to save money, time, and oftentimes saturated fat and calories if you are organized enough to have the right foods on hand. Good nutrition certainly starts in the supermarket! One trick to packing your lunch is to schedule "food shopping" into your training log. A second trick is to make lunch the night before.

The following suggestions can help you pack a super sports lunch:
- To prevent sandwich bread from getting stale, keep in it the freezer and take out the slices as needed. Bread thaws in minutes at room temperature, or in seconds in the microwave oven. Make several sandwiches at one time, and then store them in the freezer. The frozen sandwich will be thawed—and fresh—by lunchtime. Sliced turkey, lean roast beef, peanut butter, and leftover pizza freeze nicely. Don't freeze eggs, mayonnaise, jelly, lettuce, tomatoes, or raw veggies.
- Instead of eating a dry sandwich with no mayonnaise, add moistness using low-fat mayonnaise; low-fat bottled salad dressings, such as ranch or creamy Italian; mustard or ketchup; lettuce and tomato.
- Enjoy peanut butter! It is filled with health-protective fat that reduces your risk of heart disease and diabetes. Combine peanut butter (or other nut butters) with sliced banana, raisins, dates, sunflower seeds, apple slices, or celery slices.
- Add zip to a (low-fat) cheese sandwich with oregano, Italian seasonings, green peppers, and tomatoes.
- Pack leftover soups, chili, and pasta dinners for the next day's lunch. You can either eat the leftovers cold, or heat them in the office microwave oven.

Fast-Food Lunches

Because of busy schedules, few marathoners make the effort to organize their lunch plans in advance of noontime. Hence, fast foods can save the day—or they can spoil your sports diet. The good news is most quick-service restaurants now offer more low-fat foods than ever before. But, you'll still be confronted by the fatty temptations that jump out at you. Before succumbing to grease, remind yourself that you will feel better and feel better about yourself if you eat well.

Here are suggestions for some lower-fat choices:

Dunkin' Donuts: Egg white veggie flatbread, bagel, juice, chicken noodle soup, (decaf) latte light

Deli: Bagel with bean or broth-based soups; sandwiches or subs with whole-grain bread and half the filling, little or no mayonnaise (or, ask for two extra slices of bread or a second roll to make a sandwich for your second lunch with the excessive meat)

McDonald's: Grilled chicken sandwich, apple dippers, high-carb fluids such as juices, chocolate milk, hot cocoa with nonfat milk, and yes, even soft drinks (in moderation) can fuel your muscles

Wendy's: Bowl of chili with a plain baked potato

Taco Bell: Bean burrito, fresco chicken soft taco, gordita baja fresco-style.

Pizza: Thick-crust (preferably whole wheat) with extra veggies rather than extra cheese or pepperoni

Pasta: Spaghetti or ziti with tomato sauce and a glass of low-fat milk for protein; be cautious of lasagna, tortellini, or manicotti that are filled with cheese (i.e., high in saturated fat)

Chinese: Hot and sour or wonton soup; plain rice with stir-fried entrees such as beef and broccoli or chicken with pea pods; request the food be cooked with minimal oil; limit fried appetizers and fried entrees

Salad for Lunch

Salads, whether served as a main dish or an accompaniment, are a simple way to boost your intake of fresh vegetables; that's good! But as a runner, you need a substantial, carbohydrate-based lunch. Most salads get the bulk of their calories from salad oil; bad! You'll be better able to fuel your muscles if you choose a sandwich with a side salad for lunch, rather than eat just a big salad for the entire meal.

Three tricks to making a healthy sports salad are:
1. Choose a variety of colorful vegetables—dark green lettuces, red tomatoes, yellow peppers, and orange carrots—for a variety of vitamins and minerals.
2. Monitor the dressing. Some marathoners drown 50 calories of healthful salad ingredients with 400 calories of blue cheese dressing!
3. Add extra carbohydrates:
   - dense vegetables, such as corn, peas, beets, carrots
   - beans and legumes, such as chickpeas, kidney beans, and three-bean salad
   - cooked rice or pasta
   - oranges, apples, raisins, grapes, dried cranberries
   - toasted croutons
   - whole-grain bread or roll on the side

If you choose to use regular dressings, try to select ones made with olive oil for both a nice flavor and health-protective monounsaturated fats. If you want to reduce your fat intake, simply dilute regular dressings with water, more vinegar, or even milk (in ranch and other mayonnaise-based dressings). Or, choose from the plethora of low-fat and fat-free salad dressings. Low-fat dressings are good not only for salads, but also sandwiches, baked potatoes, and dips.

If the vegetables you buy for salads tend to spoil in your refrigerator before you get around to eating them all, buy smaller amounts from a salad bar at the grocery store or deli.

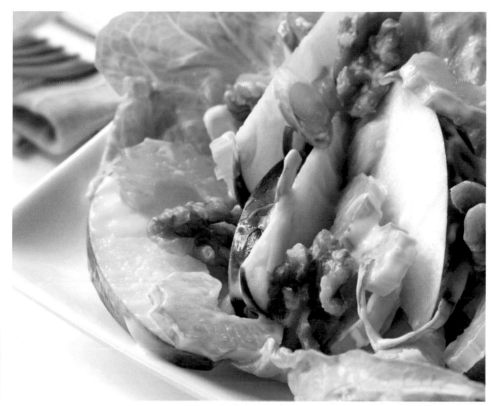

© Thinkstock/iStock

Salads

Here are how some popular salad ingredients compare. Note that the ones with the most color have the most nutritional value.

Salad Ingredient	Vitamin C (mg)	Vitamin A (IU)	Magnesium (mg)
Daily Value	*60*	*5,000*	*400*
Broccoli, 5" stalk (180 g)	110	2,500	24
Green pepper, 1/2 (70 g)	65	210	20
Spinach, 2 cups raw (110 g)	50	8,100	90
Tomato, medium (12 g)	25	760	15
Romaine, 2 cups (110 g)	30	3,000	10
Iceburg, 2 cups (110 g)	5	360	5
Cucumber, 1/2 medium (150 g)	10	325	15
Celery, 1 stalk (40 g)	5	55	4

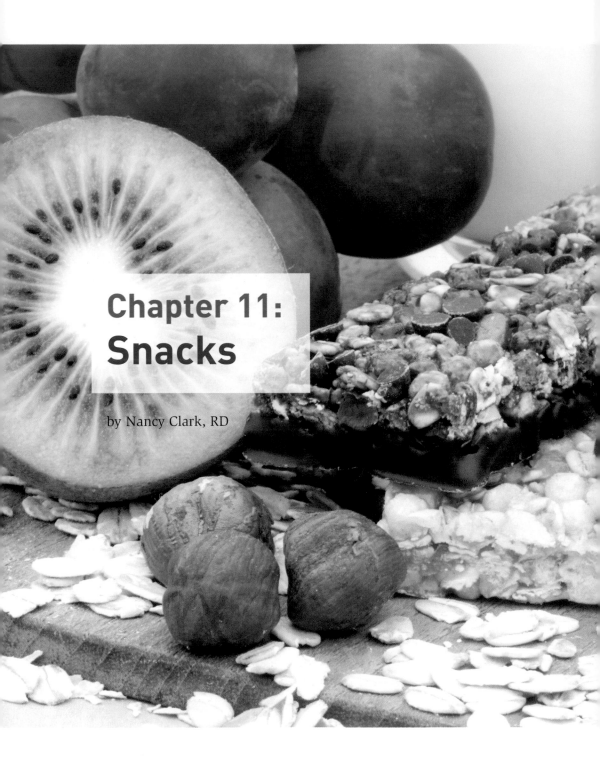

Chapter 11:
Snacks

by Nancy Clark, RD

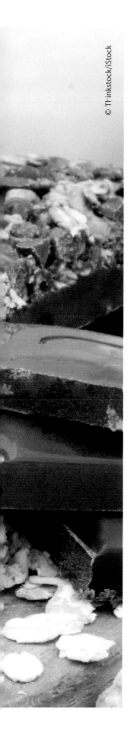

© Thinkstock/iStock

Taming the Cookie Monster

"I know I shouldn't eat cookies–but I just can't help myself. I'm a cookie monster!"

Sound familiar? Everyone knows that cookies (and candy, cakes, pies, ice cream, other sweets) offer suboptimal nutrition. But why are cookies so popular? Why do we eat monstrous portions that were not a part of our food intentions?

Why? Because cookies (and other sweets) taste good. Because athletes–and all people, for that matter–who get too hungry tend to crave sweets. Most athletes believe cookies are the problem. I challenge that belief. I see cookies as being the symptom and getting too hungry as being the problem. That is, when you get too hungry, you experience a very strong drive to eat. Cookies!!!

Hunger, A Simple Request for Fuel

Hunger is a very powerful physiological force that creates a strong desire to eat. When a child complains about being hungry, the parent readily provides food. But when athletes experience hunger, they either have "no time" to eat or, if weight-conscious, they fear food as being fattening; eating equates to getting fat.

Most athletes eat without getting fat. Food, after all, is fuel. But cookie monster problems arise when time-deprived or dieting athletes consume inadequate fuel and hunger becomes the norm. The result is an abnormal physiological state known as starvation—or more commonly known as being "on a diet." Although starvation is associated with famine in poor countries, starvation is also common among busy and dieting athletes.

In 1950, Ancel Keys and his colleagues at the University of Minnesota studied the physiology of starvation. They carefully monitored 36 young, healthy, psychologically normal men who for six months were allowed to eat only half their normal intake (similar to a very restrictive reducing diet). For three months prior to this semi-starvation diet, the researchers carefully studied each man's behaviors, personality, and eating patterns. They also observed the men for three to nine months of refeeding.

As the subjects' bodyweight fell, the researchers learned that many of the symptoms that might have been thought to be specific to binge eating were actually the result of starvation. The most striking change was a dramatic increase with food preoccupation. The hungry subjects thought about food all the time. They talked about it, read about it, dreamed about it, even collected recipes. They dramatically increased their consumption of coffee and tea and chewed gum excessively. They became depressed, had severe mood swings, experienced irritability, anger, and anxiety. They became withdrawn and lost their sense of humor. They had cold hands and feet and felt weak and dizzy. During the study, some of the men were unable to maintain control over food; they would binge eat if the opportunity presented itself—similar to breaking a diet or bingeing on cookies.

When the study ended and the men could eat freely, many of them ate continuously—big meals followed by snacks. They ate and ate—like a cookie monster. So what can we learn about binge eating from this study?

1. Preoccupation with cookies (and sweets) indicates your body is too hungry. Hunger creates a strong physiological drive to eat.
2. Cookie binges stem from starvation. If you are unable to stop eating once you start, you have likely gotten monstrously hungry (or are very stressed).
3. Dieters who restrict to the point of semi-starvation are likely to blow their diets and consequently acquire some benefits: less hunger, cookies (and other sweets), and more energy.

Living Without Hunger

In our society, people live in hunger because the prevailing messages are "I don't have time to eat" and "food is fattening." Athletes believe the best way to lose weight is to severely restrict calories. The only opportunity dieters have to eat cookies (and other tasty foods) is when they blow their diets and turn into cookie monsters. But there is another way to manage cookies:

1. Prevent hunger by eating enough at meals. You can lose weight by eating 10% to 20% fewer calories, not 50% fewer.

2. Enjoy a cookie or two as a part of an overall healthful daily food plan.

To know how many calories (and cookies) you are entitled to eat to negate hunger and manage your weight, do this simple math:

- Take your weight (or a good weight for your body) and multiply it by 10. This estimates your resting metabolic rate (RMR, the amount of energy you need to simply exist, pump blood, breathe). If you weigh 140 pounds, your RMR is about 1,400 calories—the amount you'd burn if you were to run for 14 miles!

- Add to your RMR about half that number for activities of daily living. For example, if you weigh 140 pounds and are moderately active (without your purposeful exercise), you need about 700 calories for daily living. Add fewer calories if you are sedentary.

- Next, add calories for purposeful exercise. For example, a 140 lb person would need about 1,400 calories (RMR) + 700 (daily living) + 300 (for 30 minutes of exercise) = 2,400 calories to maintain weight. To lose weight, deduct 20%, to about 1,900 calories. This translates into 600 calories for breakfast/snack, 700 for lunch/snack, and 600 for dinner/snack (or the equivalent of 11-13 Fig Newtons per section of the day).

The next time you get into a cookie frenzy, use food labels to calculate your day's intake. You'll likely see a huge discrepancy between what you have eaten and what your body deserves. No wonder you are craving cookies! Once you recognize the power of hunger, you can take steps to prevent it by eating before you get too hungry.

Living With Cookies

If you like cookies too much—to the extent you have trouble stopping eating them once you start—the way to take the power away from cookies is to eat them more often (in appropriate portions) and not try to "stay away from them." Apples likely have no "power" over you because you give yourself permsission to eat an apple whenever you want. But cookies will have power over you if you routinely restrict them. By enjoying a cookie with every lunch, you'll start to want fewer cookies. They will lose their appeal, and the cookie monster will rest in its cage, peacefully.

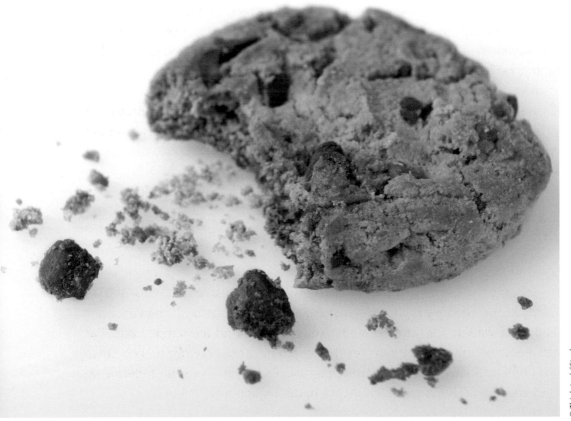

© Thinkstock/iStock

Solving the 4:00 Munchies Problem

Many runners believe eating in the afternoon is sinful. They self-inflict "Thou shalt not snack" as an Eleventh Commandment. Then, they succumb and feel guilty. As I have mentioned before, hunger is simply your body's request for fuel.

Hunger is neither bad nor wrong. It is a normal physiological function. You can expect to get hungry every four hours. For example, if you eat lunch at noon, you can appropriately be hungry by 4:00. Eat something—preferably a second lunch!

"Second lunch" conjures up visions of real food—a second sandwich, a mug of soup, or peanut butter on crackers and a (decaf) latte. In comparison, "afternoon snack" suggests candy, cookies, and sweets. Marathoners who fail to eat enough at breakfast and first lunch generally crave afternoon sweets. The preferred solution to sweet cravings is to prevent the cravings by eating more food earlier in the day.

A second lunch is particularly important for dieters. As I will discuss in chapter 17, a planned afternoon lunch of 300 to 500 calories (or whatever fits into your calorie budget) will prevent extreme hunger and reduce the risk of blowing your diet that evening.

Second Lunch Suggestions

Some runners enjoy a second sandwich for their second lunch. But others like to graze on two or three wholesome snacks from this list. If you carry snacks with you, or keep a supply of "emergency food" in your desk drawer that's ready and waiting for the 4:00 munchies, you can avoid the temptations that lurk in every convenience store, vending machine, or bakery. Try to pick items from two or three different food groups, such as carrots + cottage cheese + crackers; or graham crackers + peanut butter + apple.

Nonperishable snacks to keep stocked in your desk drawer:

- cold cereal (by the handful right out of the box or in a bowl with milk)
- hot cereal (packets of instant oatmeal are easy)
- reduced-fat microwave popcorn
- canned soup
- canned tuna
- low-fat crackers (Ak-Mak, Wasa, Melba Toast)
- graham crackers
- granola bars
- energy bars
- juice boxes or bottled juice
- dried fruit
- peanut butter or other nut butters
- nuts, trail mix

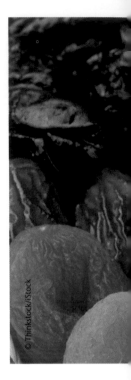

© Thinkstock/iStock

Perishable snacks to carry with you or buy fresh:

- whole-wheat bagel
- low-fat bran muffin
- microwaved potato
- Greek yogurt, low-fat
- cottage cheese, low-fat
- cheese sticks, low-fat
- hard boiled egg
- hummus and pita bread
- thick-crust pizza
- fresh fruit
- baby carrots
- leftover pasta
- frozen meal
- peanut butter sandwich

Vending machine snacks: Vending-machine cuisine offers tough choices. But tucked between the lackluster choices, you may be able to find pretzels,

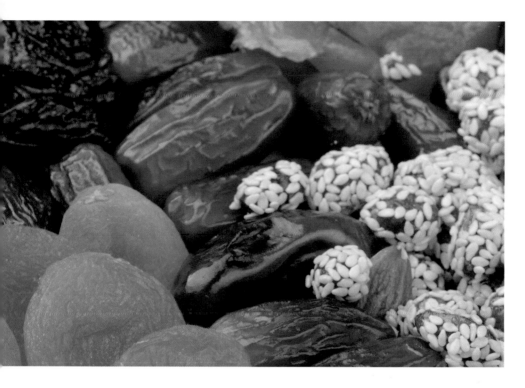

peanuts, juice, yogurt, or even an apple. The good part about vending machine snacks is that they are limited in size (e.g., only three cookies instead of the whole bag) and generally provide only 200 to 400 calories, not 2,000.

If trying to decide between fatty or sugary choices (i.e., chips vs. jelly beans), remember that the sugar in jellybeans will at least fuel your muscles, whereas the fat in the chips will clog the arteries. (After eating a sugary snack, be sure to brush or rinse your teeth.)

Cookie monster snacks: If it's cookies, brownies, an ice cream sundae, or any other such treat that you crave once a week or so, I recommend you satisfy your hankering by enjoying the treat in place of one of your lunches. Simply trade in your lunch-calories for treat-calories, so you won't be overeating. You won't destroy your health with an occasional treat, as long as your overall diet tends to be wholesome. Looking at the weekly picture, you want to target a diet that averages 90% quality foods, 10% treats.

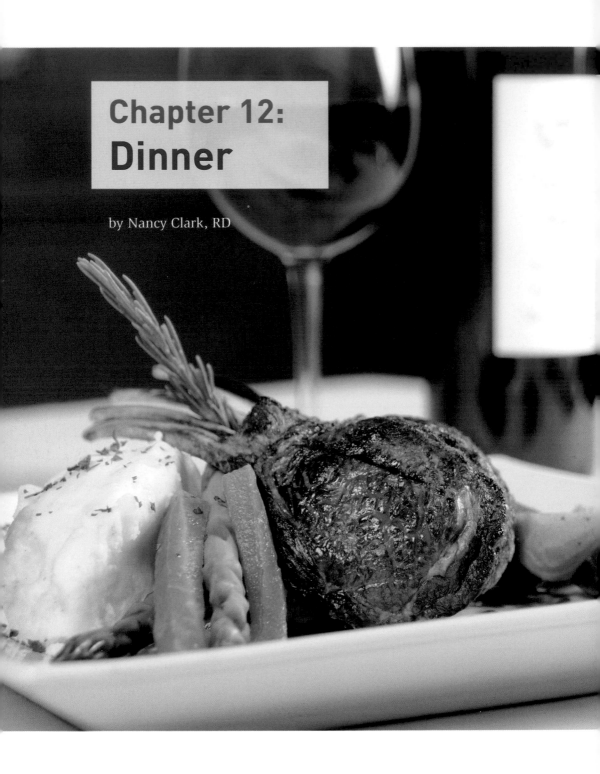

Chapter 12:
Dinner

by Nancy Clark, RD

© Thinkstock/iStock

Dinnertime generally marks the end of the workday, a time to relax and enjoy a pleasant meal—that is, if you have the energy to prepare it. The trick to dining on a balanced dinner—the protein-starch-vegetable kind that mom used to make with at least three kinds of foods—is to arrive home with enough energy to cook. This means fueling your body and brain with adequate calories prior to dinnertime—with a second lunch.

If you are far from being a master chef, you might want to take a cooking class at your local center for adult education. But no number of cooking classes will help if you arrive home too hungry to cook or make wise food choices.

Quick Fixes:
Dinner Tips for Hungry Runners

Because good nutrition starts in the supermarket, you have a far better chance of achieving a super sports diet when your kitchen is well stocked with appropriate foods. You might want to muster up your energy to marathon shop at the discount or warehouse food store once every two or three weeks and really shop, so that you have enough food to last for a while. To help accomplish this goal, post a copy of the sidebar, *Runner's Basic Shopping List,* on your refrigerator and check off the foods you need.

By keeping your kitchen well stocked with basic foods, you will have the makings for simple meals such as

- spaghetti with tomato sauce plus hamburger, ground turkey, tofu, beans, cheese cottage, grated cheese, or vegetables;
- english muffin or pita pizzas;
- tuna noodle casserole;
- soup and sandwiches (tuna, toasted cheese, peanut butter with banana);
- microwaved potato topped with cottage cheese, baked beans, or yogurt;
- peanut butter crackers and V-8 juice;
- bean burritos (frozen, or made with canned refried beans + salsa + tortilla).

Some runners use their morning shower/shave time to cook 1.5 cups of raw rice while getting ready for work. Come dinnertime, they simply brown one pound of lean hamburger or ground turkey in a large skillet, dump in the cooked rice, and then add whatever is handy. By cooking 1.5 cups or raw rice for each pound of raw lean meat, they generate two generous sports meals with 60 percent of the calories from carbohydrates.

Some popular creations with rice and ground meat include:
- Mexican—add canned beans + chili powder + grated low-fat cheddar cheese + diced tomatoes
- Chinese—add broccoli zapped in the microwave oven while the meat cooks + soy sauce
- Italian—add green beans + Italian seasonings such as basil, oregano, and garlic powder
- American—add grated low-fat Cheddar cheese + onion browned with the meat + diced tomatoes

Soup

Thick and hearty soups, abundant with carbs from rice, barley, or beans, are welcomed foods for runners. The soups' carbs refuel the muscles and the broth replaces the water and sodium lost in sweat. I like to keep soups and stews on hand for quick evening meals that simply need to be heated. A bowl of warm soup is a relatively effortless dinner, thanks to the microwave oven— and a wonderful greeting upon returning from a long winter run!

If you frequently make soups or stews, you might want to:
- Save the cooking water from vegetables in a jar in the refrigerator to use as a soup base.
- Limit the seasonings so that you can add the seasoning-of-the-day into the individual portion you will be eating. That way, you can have Chinese-style chicken soup one day, curried chicken soup another, and Mexican a third.

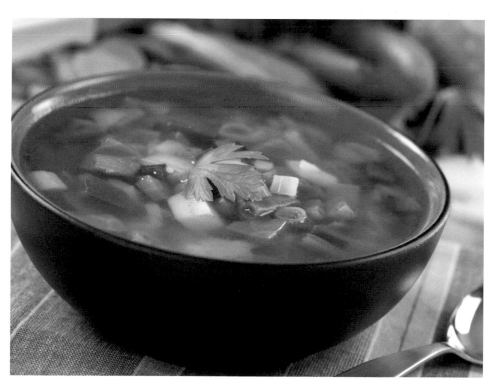

© Thinkstock/iStock

There is nothing wrong with using canned soups or broths for the foundation of a quick and easy meal. Because the canned products tend to have more sodium than do some homemade soups and stews, runners with high blood pressure should choose the low-sodium canned soups.

Here are some ways to convert plain ol' canned soup into a more exotic meal, light supper, or snack:
- Combine soups:
  onion and chicken noodle
  tomato and vegetable
- Add ingredients:
  diced celery, broccoli, tomatoes, or whatever fresh or frozen vegetable is handy
  leftover rice, noodles, pasta
  leftover vegetables, salads, casseroles
  whatever in the fridge needs to be eaten
- Add seasonings:
  curry powder to chicken soup
  cloves to tomato soup
  wine, sherry, vermouth to mushroom soup

Quick and Easy Meal Ideas

Here are some ideas for quick-and-easy meals:
- pasta with clam sauce, tomato sauce, or frozen vegetables, or low-fat cheese
- canned beans, rinsed and then spooned over rice, pasta, or salads
- frozen dinners, supplemented with whole-grain bread and fresh fruit
- Pierogies, tortellini, and burritos from the frozen food section
- baked potato topped with cottage cheese
- whole-grain cereal (hot or cold) with fruit and low-fat milk
- thick-crust pizza, fresh or frozen, then reheated in the toaster oven
- bean soups, homemade, canned, or from the deli

- quick-cooking brown rice—cook double for the next day's rice and bean salad
- stir-fry, using precut vegetables from the market, salad bar, or freezer
- Add toppings:
  Parmesan cheese
  grated low-fat cheeses
  cottage cheese
  sesame seeds
  croutons

Summary

If you are like many runners who struggle with eating well on a daily basis, you need to remember the following keys to a successful sports diet:

1. Eat appropriately sized meals at least every four hours (such as 7:00 a.m.-11:00 and 3:00-7:00 p.m.) so that you won't get too hungry. Notice how your lunches and dinner deteriorate when you eat too little breakfast and get too hungry.
2. Spend your calories on a variety of wholesome foods at each meal; target at least three kinds of food per meal.
3. Pay attention to how much better you feel, run, and feel about yourself when you eat a well-balanced sports diet.

It's my opinion that getting too hungry is the biggest problem with most runners' diets. Hearty meals based on carb-rich whole grains, fruit, and vegetables set the stage for a top-notch sports diet.

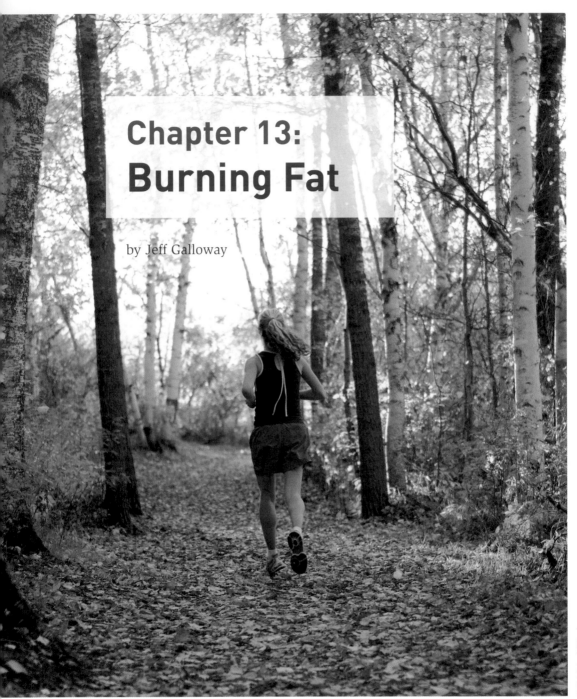

Chapter 13:
Burning Fat

by Jeff Galloway

© Thinkstock/iStock

Cognitive Eating Strategy + Gentle Exercise = Success

If you haven't read the first ten pages of this book, please do so. This sets up the concepts for fat burning and nutrition which are listed next in greater detail. Most readers find that reading the first chapter helps to give organization to the fat-burning program in this chapter.

We allow the subconscious brain (SCB) to conduct most of our activities throughout the day. The SCB is programmed to lead us to foods that contain sugar, salt, and fat, which deliver a quick dose of dopamine joy and keep the body supplied with energy and potential energy (fat). If we allow the subconscious brain to conduct our eating behaviors we can consume large quantities of calories without any accountability and are susceptible to emotional eating.

We gain control over our food and energy flow by using the executive brain in the frontal lobe to focus on choosing and accounting for each food eaten. This powerful conscious brain overrides the SBC, allowing you to make changes in diet, alter body shape, and activate other brain components that can make you into an exercising animal. As we add running, walking steps, and other exercise, we can burn off the storage that literally weighs us down.

It is possible to lose fat without running 100 miles a week or being hungry all the time. It starts with the conscious decision to be the captain of your energy ship and then setting up a strategy and a plan to make it happen. Strategy means frontal lobe control which disconnects you from emotional dopamine eating as long as you are in conscious control.

By following the strategies in this book you can lose the "last ten" or the "next ten pounds." First, here are the forces behind fat accumulation and the tools that can allow you to set up your strategy.

Concepts of Fat Burning

- The set point brain circuit is programmed to add a bit more fat every year, and to put more fat into storage when food is available.

- There are many circuits in our SBC that are triggered to eat more than we need. The resulting fat accumulation ensured survival for ancestors in prehistoric times and are powerfully embedded in our brain.

- Aerobic running, with liberal walk breaks, activates and enhances our fat burning, while reducing set point fat increase. Also remember that you must maintain a calorie deficit to lose body fat.

- Long, aerobic runs can increase the body's fat-burning capacity.

- During speed training and fast running you're not burning fat, but glycogen (stored form of carbohydrate). So slower is better for fat burning because you can go farther and burn more calories. Speed training burns calories but dramatically increases fatigue and results in fewer total workout calories burned, according to my monitoring of clients.

- Walking is aerobic—the more steps you take, the more calories you burn without a significant hunger response.

- Monitor food intake and you will activate the conscious brain—and be in control over your eating.

Tools That Help You Shift Away From SCB Emotional Eating

1. Use a website like www.fitday.com to monitor your intake and analyze your diet. Then, consult with a registered dietitian who specializes in sports nutrition to help you create a personalized plan that will help you meet your goals. The referral network at www.scandpg.org can help you find a local nutrition professional.

2. Use a resource like this book or *Running and Fatburning for Women* by Barbara and Jeff Galloway or Nancy Clark's *Sports Nutrition Guidebook* for back-up information—and to understand the process.

3. Create just a small (but sustainable) calorie deficit goal each day (150-250 recommended).

4. Stay within your calorie budget for each day.

5. Get a step counter and increase the number of walking steps to achieve your calorie deficit (10,000 steps is the goal).

6. As you monitor your eating and exercise, you gain control and can take action to improve efficiency of the process. You are in command over your budget.

How to Modify Reflex Eating Behaviors

- Estimate calorie content before eating anything—this shifts consciousness to frontal lobe.
- If there are foods that you really love, which are hazardous to your calorie budget, eat small amounts on a regular basis and account for them.
- Search for foods that are healthy that you can gradually swap for the hazard foods.
- Reward yourself for making progress with non-food items.

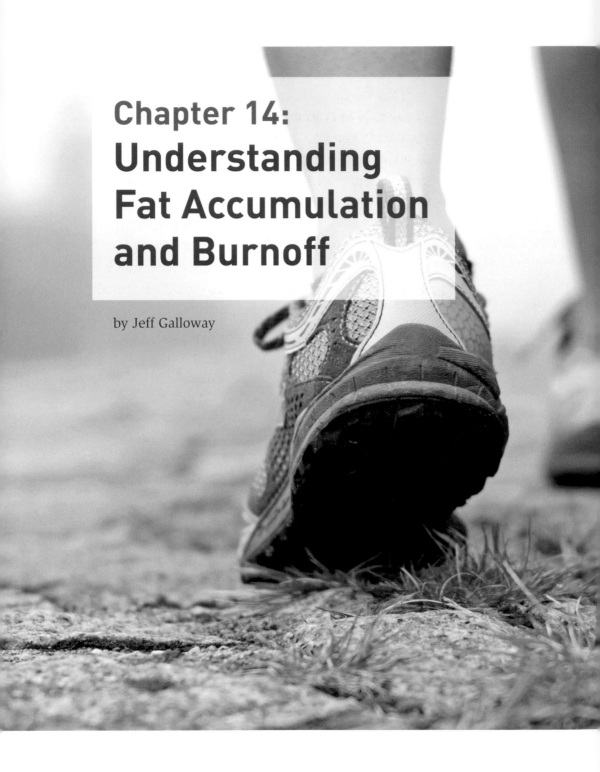

Chapter 14:
Understanding Fat Accumulation and Burnoff

by Jeff Galloway

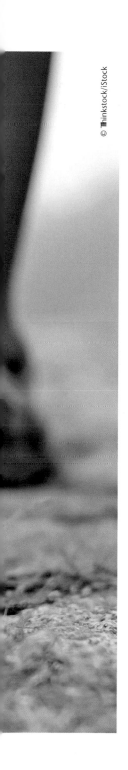

© Thinkstock/iStock

Fat is our genetic insurance policy against starvation and prolonged sickness, which were real threats for our ancestors during millions of years of evolution. Fat is the efficient fuel your body can use during endurance exercise. A powerful brain circuit evolved, the "set point", to promote continual fat storage when food was available. This fat storage allowed individuals to survive regular periods of starvation, prolonged sickness, and injury. The set point is programmed to increase a bit more accumulation as the years go by—so it's natural to weigh more at 47 than you did at 37. But there is hope for those who want to lose some of this "insurance." By learning how to budget calories you can enjoy foods as you gain control over your fat accumulation and reduce storage.

Reducing food intake by itself is not the fun part of lowering fat levels—nor is it a successful strategy over the long term. While going on a "diet" (reducing the amount of food consumed) can definitely result in a bodyweight reduction, this is almost always a temporary situation. Food deprivation activates what we call the *starvation reflex* which stimulates a "rebound" in fat accumulation once the diet is over. While creating a calorie deficit is the best way to lose undesired body fat, exercise is the best way to keep it off. By increasing gentle exercise as you control consumption you set up a successful process that is sustainable. Best part is that with exercise, you don't have to be hungry all the time—as you would be if you were on a starvation diet.

The right exercise, at the right exertion level can bring joy to your life. If you haven't experienced this, you haven't been doing it right. In chapter 19, you'll find a fat reduction training schedule that is gentle, has a number of options, and burns fat without pain. When exercise is right for you, a positive attitude and a glow is bestowed by every session—you want to come back and do it again. Exercise gives you more energy for your day, a positive attitude, and erases or controls stress build-up while it revs up the furnace that can burn off the potential energy in storage.

With this plan you are eating often, regularly moving yourself, and becoming an active person involved in life. This gives you the energy to think clearly, perform your daily activities, and enjoy family and life. You're in control.

How does fat accumulate?

Eating more calories than are burned off, day after day, promotes fat deposition.

The set point ensured survival of the species.

After millions of years of evolution, the bodies we have inherited have been programmed to hold on to the fat you have stored because this ensured survival of the species. Before humans understood disease and food storage, our ancestors were susceptible to sweeping infections and starvation. Those who had above average fat stores survived periods of starvation and sickness, and passed on the fat accumulation adaptation to their children. The replication of this process over thousands of generations has resulted in the powerful **set point**.

This biologically engineered survival mechanism is programmed to increase the fat storage levels each year. Changing the set point puts you into a confrontation with a process that has been in place for over millions of years, making you the underdog. It is possible to reduce fat levels, but you must set realistic goals for fat management.

The lowest set point is experienced in the early 20s.

Many experts agree that by about the age of 25 we have accumulated a level of fat that the body intuitively marks as its lowest level. This set point is programmed to increase a little each year. The amount of increase is so small in the 20s and early 30s, that we usually don't realize that we're adding it— until about 10 years later, when it's time to go to a class reunion.

Humans are supposed to carry around fat. But your set point does too good a job, continuing to add to the percentage, each year, every year. And the amount of increase seems to be significantly greater as we get older. Even when you've had a year when stress or illness prevented the usual increase, the set point has memory and makes up by increasing appetite more than normal during the following year or two. Go ahead, shout "Unfair!" as loud as you wish. Your set point doesn't argue, it just makes another deposit. There is hope: Exercise has allowed many to manage it.

Men and women deposit fat differently.

While men tend to deposit fat on the surface of the skin, women (particularly in their 20s and 30s) fill up internal storage areas first. Young women use the "pinch test" to check fat levels and aren't concerned until the hidden fat areas are somewhat full and the fat spills on to the surface of the body. For more information in this area, see *Fit or Fat?* by biochemist Dr. Covert Bailey.

A common woman's complaint in the 30s or early 40s is the following: "My body has betrayed me—just during the past year I've been adding fat." In fact, fat has been deposited at a fairly consistent rate but hidden from view for many years. With many women, it is only when the internal fat storage areas are filled that they notice surface fat build-up.

Men find it easier to burn fat than women.

When men start exercising regularly, many lose fat and weight for several months. Probably related to biological issues, and primitive protections for mothers, women have a harder time burning it off. The reality is that you are ahead of the others in our society…even if you are *maintaining* the same weight. A 45-year-old woman in the US can easily gain two to three pounds a year. Regular gentle exercise (including strategic longer runs and taking more walking steps throughout the day) commonly allows women to hold the set point steady for years, and this is a victory. In other words, the set point may be controlled even if you are holding at the same weight, year to year.

Restrictive diets don't work because of the starvation reflex.

We are certainly capable of lowering food intake for days, weeks, and months to lower fat levels and weight. This is a form of starvation, and the set point has a long-term memory. Let's say that we lose 10 pounds by a calorie restrictive diet during the two months before the class reunion. When the diet ends, you'll experience a starvation reflex: a slight increase in appetite and hunger over weeks and months until the fat accumulated on your body is higher than it was before the diet. It's a fact that almost all of those who lose fat on a diet put more pounds back (than they lost) within months of diet termination.

Waiting too long to eat triggers the starvation reflex.

If you are hungry and wait more than three hours without eating something, your set point organism senses that you may be going into a period of starvation. (*Fit or Fat?* by Dr. Covert Bailey) The longer you wait to eat, the more you will feel these three effects of the starvation reflex:

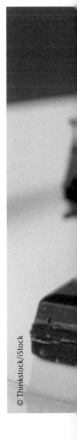

© Thinkstock/iStock

1. A reduction in your metabolism rate: drowsy, lazy, no energy. Imagine an internal voice saying something like this, "If this person is going to start depriving me of food I had better tune down the metabolism rate to conserve resources." A slower metabolism means that you have little or no energy to exercise or move around.

2. An increase in the fat-depositing enzymes. The longer you wait to eat something, the more enzymes you will have, and the more fat will be actually deposited from your next meal.

3. Your appetite increases. The longer you wait to eat, the more likely it is that, for the next few meals, you will have an increased appetite: You're still hungry after a normal meal.

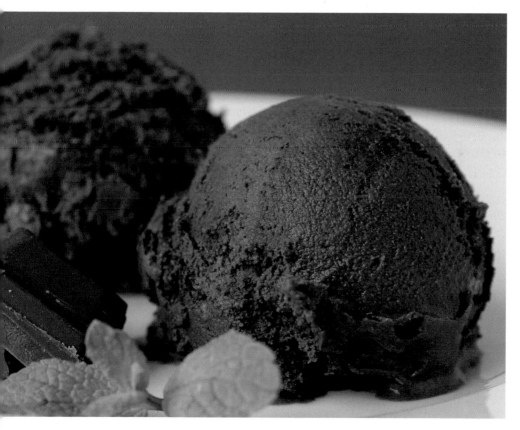

True Ice Cream Confessions (From Jeff)

(An example of the starvation reflex)

Barbara and I used to like a particular type of ice cream so much that we ate a quart or more of it, several nights a week. It was the reward we gave ourselves for reaching exercise goals for that day. Then, on a fateful New Year's Day, we decided to eliminate the chocolate chip mint ice cream from our diet—after more than 10 years of enjoyment. We were successful for two years. A leftover box after a birthday party got us re-started on the habit, and we even increased our intake over what it had been before—due to having deprived ourselves.

You can "starve" yourself of a food that you dearly love for an extended period of time. But at some time in the future, when the food is around and no one else is...you will tend to over-consume that food.

Jeff's correction for this problem was the following:

1. I made a contract with myself: I could have a little of it whenever I wanted—while promising to be reasonable.
2. Setting a goal of enjoying one bowl a week, five years from now.
3. Four years from now, enjoying a bowl every five days.
4. Three years from now, a bowl every four days.
5. Learning to enjoy healthy sweet things, like fruit salads and energy bars, as replacements.

It worked! I hardly ever eat any ice cream... but sometimes enjoy a bowl if I want. This is purely for medicinal reasons, you understand.

Low-carb diets can be a scam.

Low-carb diets produce, primarily, a water weight loss—not a fat loss. The lack of sufficient carbohydrate causes a relatively quick loss of 4-10 pounds due to not restocking the glycogen (fuel stored in the muscle that is needed for exercise). For every gram of glycogen, there are 2.5 grams of water stored nearby to burn the glycogen. When the glycogen storage goes away, so does the water (3-6 pounds). The fat and extra protein in low-carb diets usually adds fat to the body during the low-carb diet, but this is not noticed because the water weight loss is registered by the scales. When the dieter goes back to eating carbohydrate again, the water and glycogen weight returns and the added fat is then noticed with a weight gain.

This is a type of starvation diet. I've heard from countless low-carb victims who admit that while they were on the diet, their psychological deprivation of carbs produced a significant rebound effect when they began eating them again. The cravings for bread, pastries, french fries, soft drinks, and other pound-adding foods, increased for months after they went off the diet. The weight goes back on, and on, and on.

- Dieting usually triggers the starvation reflex—eating small meals frequently burns more calories (*Fit or Fat?* by Dr. Covert Bailey).
- Caffeine helps in fat burning—but don't take it if you have problems with caffeine. But you must maintain an overall calorie deficit to lose body fat.
- Find foods that make you feel satisfied, with moderate-, or lower-calorie content.

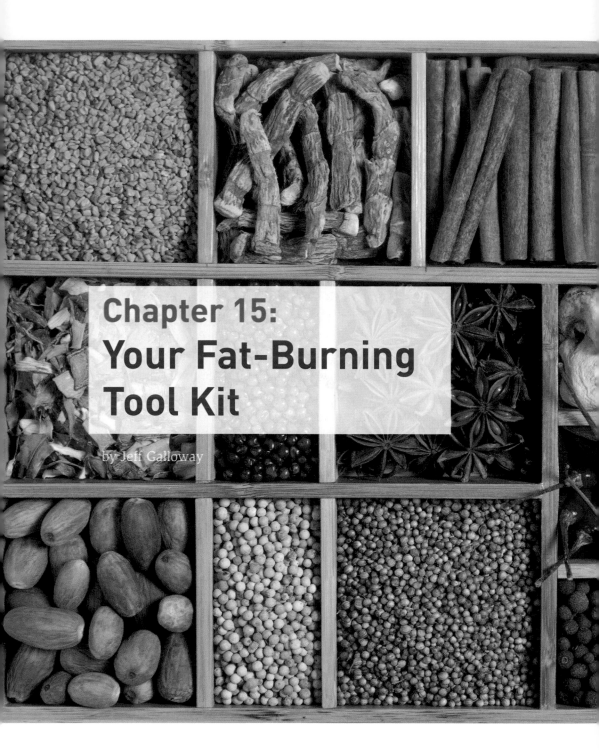

Chapter 15:
Your Fat-Burning Tool Kit

by Jeff Galloway

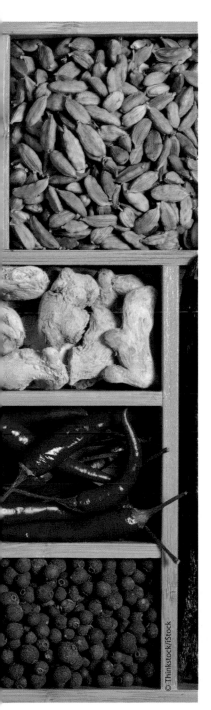

© Thinkstock/iStock

These simple tools will give you control over the fat-burning process.

BMI—Body mass index (BMI) is a fairly reliable indicator of body fat for most people and is calculated using a person's weight and height. www.cdc.gov

BMI is a calculation that allows most people to monitor fat increase or reduction, telling them whether they are gaining mass or losing it, and whether their body is "normal" sized, overweight, or obese. But take note that "most people" does not include muscular people. For example the BMI of body builders and football players can put them in the obese category, but they simply have a large body mass due to extra muscle, not extra fat. Many large runners have a BMI that labels them as obese, even though they have lost a lot of weight. They are currently lean given their genetics; they simply have a significant amount of muscle mass.

Websites or nutritional analysis-Programs, such as Weight Watchers and websites and software such as www.fitday.com, www.LoseIt. com, and www.supertracker.USDA.gov provide guidance in monitoring the income side of the calorie equation, with nutritional "reality checks." These tools help you budget your calories each day to feel satisfied, have more energy, and avoid extra intake. They also tell you whether you are getting the quantities of vitamins and minerals that you need each day.

115

Step counters—This is an almost unlimited opportunity to burn calories all day. More steps mean more calories burned. The greatest opportunity for burning calories is in adding steps to your day—walking instead of sitting. Checking your count several times a day can motivate you to add a few more here and there. It adds up quickly. Go to a technical running store and pick a quality product (usually less than $38).

Steps Add Up!

Most of the runners I've worked with find that, when walking, they can take about 100 steps a minute. So while waiting 10 minutes for a meeting to start you can get in 1,000 steps. While watching the kids play on a playground for 30 minutes, another 3,000 steps are added to your calorie-burning side of the ledger if you want the extra steps to contribute to fat loss. Note that you need to maintain a calorie deficit to burn fat.

Bathroom scale—Weigh in immediately after getting out of bed and going to the bathroom. This is a general guide but not exact. There are lots of fluctuations due to fluid levels from day to day. You have to run about 35 miles to burn a pound of fat. If you lost 3 pounds from one morning to the next, and you didn't run 105 miles the day before, the major cause of weight loss was fluid changes—often dehydration or carbohydrate restriction. I suggest using the scale to show long-term weight loss. Don't be obsessed with day-to-day changes.

Shoes—Pick a pair that is comfortable and supportive for the type of foot that you have. See the Running Store Visit chapter in my other books for specific information.

A journal—Choose one that is small enough to take with you, while having space to jot down food, steps, and other exercise.

A piece of ribbon—To track the reduction of your waist.

BMI can monitor changes in body size.

One way to see how you compare to "normal weight" bodies of your same height is by computing your BMI.

Adult BMI formula:

Inches/pounds: (weight in pounds) divided by (height in inches, squared) times 703

Example:

100 pound person that is 5 feet tall—100 divided by 3600 x 703 = 19.52 BMI

Example:

200 pound person that is 5 feet tall—200 divided by 3600 x 703 = 39.05

Meters/kilograms: (weight in kilograms) divided by (height in meters, squared)

Example: 100 kilogram person that is 2 meters tall—100 divided by 4 = 25

Example: 160 kilogram person that is 2 meters tall—160 divided by 4 = 40

- Below 25 is considered "Normal"
- Adults with a BMI of 25 to 29.9 are considered "overweight".
- When the BMI exceeds 30, the classification changes to obese.

(Parents should consult with the child's pediatrician before computing BMI.)

*A kilogram is 2.2 pounds
*3.27 feet equal one meter

Another effective tool is to simply take measurements with a tape measure. Your clothes are another judge of weight loss. If you pants are looser, there is less of you! You can also look in a mirror. If you see less fat, you have less fat.

Websites and Nutritional Analysis Programs

To stay in control over the weight reduction process, you need to monitor calorie and nutritional intake. This keeps you in the frontal lobe and away from the emotional eating patterns that are hardwired into our subconscious brain.

You can choose from a variety of websites, apps, or hands-on programs (such as Weight Watchers) that offer more support. In either case, you must keep a journal of the food eaten each day: food type or brand and quantity. This report is either logged into a website or reported at the weekly meeting of the program. We have used www.fitday.com programs, both online and the software. Other sites are www.sparkpeople.com and www.calorieking.com. These services not only give you a running tally of calories in/out, but also note deficiencies of calcium, iron, B vitamins, and protein.

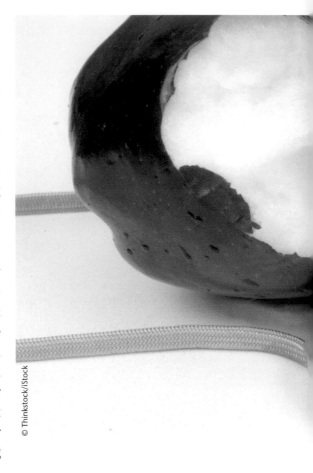

© Thinkstock/iStock

Your best bet, however, is to get personalized advice by meeting one-on-one with a sports nutritionist who can help create a program that is tailored to your needs, your lifestyle, and your food preferences. To find a local sports nutritional professional, use the referral network at www.SCANdog.org.

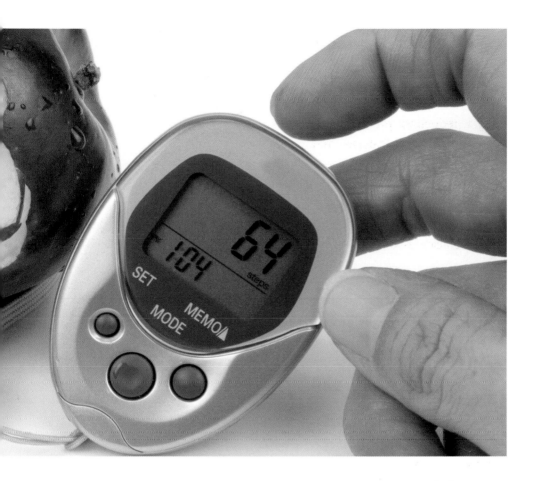

Step Counter

Not all step counters are created equal. Many are so inconsistent that you could have four of the same brand on your belt, and have four significantly different totals at day's end—sometimes thousands of steps different. It helps to get guidance from a technical running store before buying. Price range for a reliable unit is usually $25-$35. Clip it on your belt and write down the total at the end of the day. Your goal is to register more than 10,000 a day. Every time you take a step, you're burning calories. This instrument tells you how much you're burning. There are a number of electronic devices, such as Fitbit that can wirelessly download your data to your computer for quick updates.

Bathroom Scale

Most scales tend to be reliable. We suggest doing an internet search to see which scales may be more reliable than others. For our purposes, you only need to record the weight. Immediately after rising in the morning, weigh yourself and write down the result.

Scale readings can be frustrating because even the best scales will show ups and downs for seemingly no reason. You should look at the trends. Don't get discouraged if the scales don't seem to be cooperating. There will be some days when the scales are up, even when you've increased exercise and reduced calorie intake. If you stay focused on your plan of managing the income and increasing or maintaining exercise level, you will be rewarded. When you increase exercise, you may experience an initial weight gain that is healthy and will help you exercise easier and better (more blood volume, more glycogen for fuel).

Standardize your weight measurement and do it regularly. Some people like to weight themselves each day, others once a week or once a month. Use the same scale and weigh yourself right after you waken, before eating or drinking anything. Keep a chart and write down the weight immediately.

Shoes

Shoes are designed to support the way your foot walks or runs. The trained staff at a really good running store in your area can advise you. But first, read the shoe selection chapter in the back of this book.

Journal

This does not have to be a technical product. It should be small enough to carry in a purse or pocket. Studies show that those who write down what they eat tend to reduce the number of calories consumed. When you eat anything, write down the food, quantity or weight, and composition if available or needed. You can also record the number of steps taken each day, the type and duration of other exercise, and any other facts that can help you account for the income/expenditure of calories.

A Piece of Ribbon

Use a piece of light colored ribbon. When you start your fat-burning program, put the ribbon around the smallest section of your waist, usually slightly above your belly button or navel. Mark it, and note the date. Once a month, take out the ribbon, measure and mark with the date.

Quick Check by the Numbers
Make a chart on your wall and track the data, every six months.
- Weight
- BMI
- Resting heart rate
- Cholesterol
- HDL
- LDL
- Blood sugar—diabetes

Chapter 16:
The Calorie Budget

by Nancy Clark, RD

Many marathoners are on the "see food diet;" they see food and they eat it. They can naturally regulate a proper calorie intake and have little need to calculate calories. They simply eat when they are hungry and stop when they are content. But other marathoners see food and try to not eat it. They deem food as "fattening" and counter to their desires to be leaner, lighter runners. They have lost touch with their body's natural ability to regulate an appropriate food intake. They often do not eat when they are hungry (such as happens with severe reducing diets or skipping meals) and then overeat later in the day.

As a marathoner, you should eat your calories evenly throughout the day, not in a crescendo. That is, don't skimp on daytime meals only to spend your whole calorie budget in the evening! The better bet is to budget your calories so you eat enough at breakfast and lunch to support both an active life and a serious training program.

Eating (wholesome) calories evenly throughout the day invests in high energy, added stamina, strength, and smooth running, to say nothing of better health. If you struggle with energy lags, you might wonder how many calories are OK to eat to boost energy yet not "get fat." Knowing your calorie budget can help you estimate how much food is appropriate to:

- eat at each meal so you can avoid energy lags.
- fuel-up and refuel from workouts.
- lose desired weight and maintain energy for running.
- feel energetic, train better, and feel good about your eating.

A calorie-awareness approach to eating can help you eat the right amount of food at the right times. For example, if you skip breakfast and lunch (i.e., eat zero calories, zero fuel), you can clearly see why you lack energy for your afternoon training session. If you are weight-conscious, calorie information allows you to determine how much food you can eat for fuel yet still lose body fat.

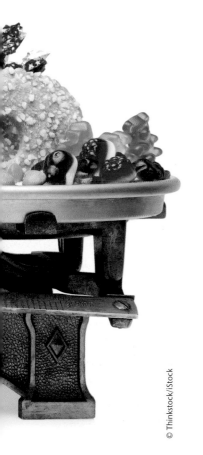

© Thinkstock/iStock

Calculating Your Calorie Needs

If you struggle with eating intuitively and want to try working with a calorie budget, here is an easy formula to help you estimate your calorie needs. For more personalized advice, I highly recommend you consult with a registered dietitian who specializes in sports nutrition. Visit the American Dietetic Association's referral networks at www.eatright.org and www.SCANdpg.org to find a local sports dietitian.

1. To estimate your resting metabolic rate (RMR), that is, the amount of calories you need to simply breathe, pump blood, and be alive:

Multiply your weight (or a good weight for your body) by 10 calories per pound (or 22 calories per kilogram).

_____weight (lbs) x 10 calories/lb = _____ calories for your RMR

Example: If you weigh 120 pounds, you need approximately 1,200 calories (120 x 10) to simply do nothing all day except exist. If you are significantly overweight, use an adjusted weight: the weight that is halfway between your desired weight and your current weight.

2. Add more calories for daily activity—apart from your running and other purposeful exercise.

* 50% x RMR if you are moderately active throughout the day
* ~30-40% if you are sedentary
* ~60-70% if you are very active (apart from your running or walking)

50% x _____RMR = _____ calories for daily activity

Example: A moderately active 120-pound woman who requires 1,200 calories for her resting metabolic rate needs about 600 more calories for activities of daily living. This totals 1,800 calories per day—without running.

3. Add more calories for your purposeful exercise. The general rule of thumb is 100 calories per mile, but more precisely, this depends upon your weight.

Body weight Calories (per mile)
lbs (kg)
120 (55) 95
140 (64) 110
160 (73) 125
180 (82) 140

____exercise calories + ____daily activity + ____RMR = ____total calories

Example: A 120-pound woman who runs five miles per day burns about 475 calories while running. This brings her to about 2,275 calories per day to maintain her weight (475 running + 600 moderate daily activity + 1,200 RMR = 2.275). For simplicity, let's just say 2,300 calories.

Note: After a very hard workout or long run, marathoners tend to rest, recover and burn fewer calories than usual during the rest of their day. Observe if this happens with you. That is, do you tend to sit more than usual—reading more or watching more TV—after having done a long weekend run? If so, adjust your calorie needs accordingly!

4. To lose weight, target 80 to 90% of total calorie needs.

80% x _____total calories = _____ calories to reduce weight

Example:
.80 x 2,300 calories = 1,840 calories, or more simply 1,800 calories/day
.90 x 2,300 calories = 2,070 calories, or more simply 2,100 calories/day

5. Now, take your calorie budget and divide it into three or four parts of the day.

For the 120-pound woman on a diet, this comes to:
Calories
Breakfast/snack 600-700 OR Breakfast 500
Lunch/snack 600-700 or Lunch 500-600
Dinner/snack 600-700 or Lunch #2 300-400
Dinner 500-600

The next step is to read food labels and get calorie information from websites (www.fitday.com, www.calorieking.com) to become familiar with the calorie content of the foods you commonly eat and then fuel your body according to the rules for a well-balanced diet.

Honor Hunger

I commonly hear marathoners complain, "Ever since I started training longer distances, I've been hungry all the time." They often feel confused by hunger and sometimes even feel guilty they are always eager to eat. One walker perceived her hunger as being bad and wrong.

Hunger is normal; it is essential for survival. Without hunger, we would waste away. Hunger is simply your body's way of requesting fuel. Hunger signals include needless fatigue, inability to focus and concentrate on the task at hand, moodiness, and cold hands and feet. These signals happen prior to a growling stomach, at which point you are too hungry.

The more you exercise, the hungrier you will get and the more fuel you will need. Plan to fuel up or refuel at least every four hours. You should not spend your day feeling hungry—even if you are on a reducing diet. (see chapter 15). If your 8:00 a.m. breakfast finds you hungry earlier than noon, your breakfast simply contained too few calories. You need a supplemental midmorning snack or a bigger breakfast that supplies about one-third of your day's calories.

Come noontime, instead of thinking something is wrong with you because you are hungry again, enjoy lunch as being the second-most-important meal of the day. Morning runners, in particular, need a hearty lunch to refuel their muscles; afternoon runners need a respectable lunch and afternoon snack/second lunch to fuel their after-work training.

Whereas some runners like to satisfy their appetites with big meals, others prefer to divide their calories into mini-meals eaten every two hours. Eat however suits your training schedule and lifestyle. But whatever you do, eat when you are physically hungry. Hunger is simply your body's request for fuel. (The next chapter offers strategies for managing food that is misused as a "drug" to calm and reward yourself; keep reading!)

Summary

Just as you know how much money you can spend when you shop, some marathoners find it helpful to know how many calories they can enjoy spending when they eat. Weight-conscious marathoners, in particular, tend to undereat during the day and overeat at night. By targeting an appropriate (and often larger than normal) breakfast and lunch, you can fuel yourself evenly throughout the day. Learn to listen to your huger cues and respond by eating appropriately sized meals and snacks. Calorie-counting can be a tool to get in touch with how much is OK to eat, but calorie-counting should become needless as you relearn how to eat intuitively.

Chapter 17:
The Eating Plan—
Meal by Meal

by Barbara Galloway

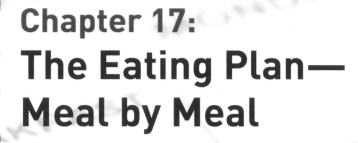

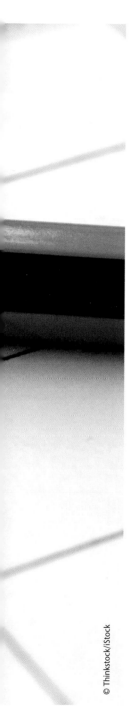

© Thinkstock/iStock

Jeff and I are your food coaches. We are not certified dietitians. We will offer strategies for getting control over eating, consuming energizing meals all day long, and expending energy all day long. Nancy Clark, who is a registered dietitian (RD), has information in her chapters in this book and in her *Sports Nutrition Guidebook*. For research-oriented evidence-based information, we highly recommend her books and articles. She does a great job of translating the science of fueling into practical, how-to food suggestions.

Choices

The following chart has only some of the many options available. Most people like to choose one item during each time period. As you log in the food consumed, you will learn how of each food much you can eat to stay within budget or adjust other items. The website of your choice will also tell you whether you are getting the daily amount of protein, calcium, fruits, vegetables, grains, and fiber that you need. Look at the labels on each product and put one portion in your bowl or on your plate. Remember to drink at least 12 oz of water during and after each meal or snack to feel more satisfied. Increased fiber content may also provide a longer feeling of satisfaction.

Note: When eating six to nine times a day, you will need to cut the portion size of some featured items. Put the extra amount into a container in the refrigerator for use as another snack later so that you don't have to prepare it.

Early Morning (300-400 Calories)

- Whole-grain bread made into French toast with fruit yogurt, juice, or frozen juice concentrate as syrup
- Whole-grain pancake with fruit and yogurt
- A portion of Grape Nuts cereal, skim milk, nonfat yogurt, and fruit
- A portion of **Barbara's special oatmeal** with a 4-oz glass of orange juice
  - ½ cup oatmeal cooked (rolled or steel cut)
  - ¼ cup skim milk
  - ½ oz walnuts
  - 1 tbs dried fruit
  - 2 tsp brown sugar or 1 tsp of molasses

Calorie count:
- Total calories: **420**
- Fat calories: 110—12 g
- Carbohydrate: 270—67 g
- Protein: 45—11 g
- Fiber: 6 g

Eggs and toast with fruit
- 2 eggs (egg beaters or eggland's best)
- 2 slices of whole-grain bread
- 4 oz orange juice
- 1 banana, or a medium apple, or a medium orange

Calorie count:
- Total **455**
- Fat: 95—11 g
- Carbohydrate: 270—66 g
- Protein: 70—19 g
- Fiber: 5 g

Mavis Lindgren's 8-grain power breakfast

Mavis was a sickly child and adult who started to exercise in her late 50s and did not have even a cold for decades. She was a wonderful person, ran marathons into her late 80s and gave us this recipe.

- 1 cup wheat berries—cook 2-3 minutes in boiling water, store in bowl with enough cool water to cover
- In a separate cooking pot:
  - 5 ½ cups of boiling water with 1 tsp of salt in water
  - ½ cup rolled oats
  - ¼ cup each: millet, rolled rye, whole-grain brown rice, rolled soy, 1 tsp flaxseed
  - Bring to a boil and simmer for 10 minutes (in double boiler if possible). Let stand overnight.
- Next morning, fold in wheat berries and serve with milk, topped with sunflower seeds, banana, dates, peanuts, granola, or whatever you want.

Cereal with milk and fruit
- 1 serving of Kelloggs Smart Start Healthy Heart cereal
- ½ cup skim milk
- 1 banana
- ½ cup skim milk
- 1 tsp Hershey's Chocolate Syrup (optional, 50 calories)

Calorie count
- Total: **400**
- Fat: 10—1 g
- Carbohydrate: 330—84 g
- Protein: 50—12 g
- Fiber: 6 g

Mid-Morning (150-200 Calories)

- Nonfat cottage cheese with fruit
- Whole-grain bread or bagel
- Fat-free yogurt with nuts and fruit
- A small bowl of whole-grain cereal with fruit
- An energy bar

Noon (400 Calories)

- Tuna fish sandwich, whole-grain bread, fat-free mayo, cole slaw (with fat-free dressing)
- Turkey breast sandwich with salad, mustard or ketchup, or fat-free mayo, celery, carrots
- Veggie burger on whole-grain bread, fat-free mayo, salad of choice
- Spinach salad with peanuts, sunflower seeds, almonds, low-fat cheese, nonfat dressing, whole-grain rolls or croutons
- Soup and salad
- 1 cup soup, example: Veggie Black Bean
- 1 cup tortilla chips—low fat

Salad: 2 cups mixed salad greens
- 4 cherry tomatoes
- 4 cucumber slices
- 2 rings, bell pepper
- 3 baby carrots
- 2 tsp low-fat salad dressing
- 12 oz non-sweetened tea or a diet drink

Calorie count
- Total: **340**
- Fat: 110—12 g
- Carbohydrate: 200—50 g
- Protein: 30—9 g
- Fiber—10 g

© Thinkstock/Monkey Business

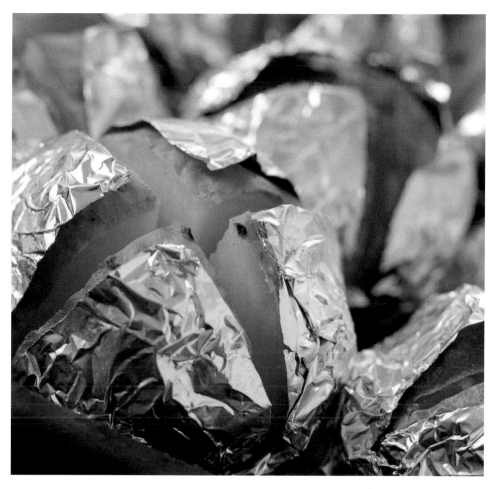

Baked potato with veggie chile

- 1 medium baked potato about 3 in diameter
- 1 lemon (vitamin C) to flavor the potato
- 1 cup veggie chili with beans (Hormel)

Calorie count:

- Total: **400**
- Fat: 10—1 g
- Carbohydrate: 330—83 g
- Protein: 60—15 g
- Fiber: 15 g

Mid-Afternoon (150-200 Calories)

- Microwave cup of soup
- ½ peanut butter sandwich—one slice of whole-grain bread with peanut butter
- Energy bar
- Small salad and one cup of fat-free cottage cheese

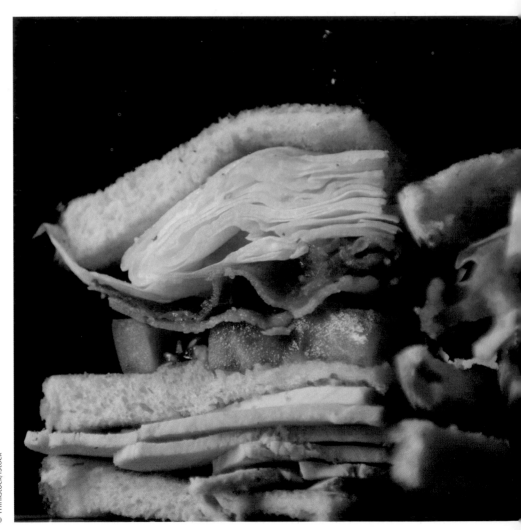

© Thinkstock/iStock

Turkey sandwich (recommend cutting in half, and refrigerating the other half for the next day)

- 3 oz of turkey breast slices
- 2 slices of whole-wheat bread
- 2 tsp of low-fat mayo
- 1 oz Swiss cheese (1 slice)
- 4 spinach leaves
- 1 tomato slice

Calorie count (based upon a whole sandwich)

- Total: **480**
- Fat: 200—25 g
- Carbohydrate: 120—30 g
- Protein: 160—41 g
- Fiber: 4 g

Peanut butter sandwich with apple and milk

- 1 slice of whole-grain bread
- 1 tbs peanut butter
- 1/2 medium size apple, sliced
- 1/2 cup, skim milk

Calorie count:

- Total: **285**
- Fat: 80—9 g
- Carbohydrate: 140—36 g
- Protein: 50—13 g
- Fiber: 6 g

Pre-Workout Snack (150 Calories)

- Energy Bar
- Toast with honey or jam (no butter or margarine)
- Cup of coffee
- ...or, if you did not eat the pre-workout snack and are a bit hungry, drink about 100-150 calories of a sports drink or juice

Post-Workout Snack (Within 30 to 60 Minutes of Finishing 100-200 Calorie)

- 200 calories of a sports recovery drink
- An energy bar that has less than 15% of the calories in fat

Dinner (400-500 Calories)

There are lots of great recipes in publications such as *Cooking Light*, and websites such as www.epicurous.com and www.allrecipes.com. The basics are listed next. What makes the meal come alive are the seasonings which are listed in the recipes. You can use a variety of fat substitutes.

- Fish or lean chicken breast or tofu (or other protein source) with whole-wheat pasta, and steamed vegetables
- Rice with vegetables and a protein source
- Dinner salad with lots of different vegetables, nuts, lean cheese, or turkey, or fish, or chicken or tofu

Chicken or tofu kabob with brown rice and cooked spinach
- 4 oz chicken breast or tofu
- 1 cup cooked brown rice
- 1 cup cooked spinach
- Pam or similar spray

Calorie count:
- Total: **500**
- Fat: 115—13 g
- Carbohydrate: 215—29 g
- Protein: 170—44 g
- Fiber: 8 g

Gazpacho

Our friend Linda Kappel gave us this recipe which can be eaten with some whole-grain bread.

- 1 clove garlic
- ½ small onion
- 1 stalk celery
- ½ small green pepper
- 3 large tomatoes, peeled
- 1 medium cucumber, peeled
- ½ cups tomato or vegetable juice
- tsp wine vinegar
- tsp olive oil
- 1 ½ tsp salt
- ½ tsp dried basil
- ¼ tsp pepper
- dash tabasco

Place all ingredients (in order listed) into food processor. Process on high speed until desired consistency. Chill.

After Dinner Snacks (50-100 Calories)

- Popcorn
- A piece of chocolate
- A glass of wine
- A glass of water

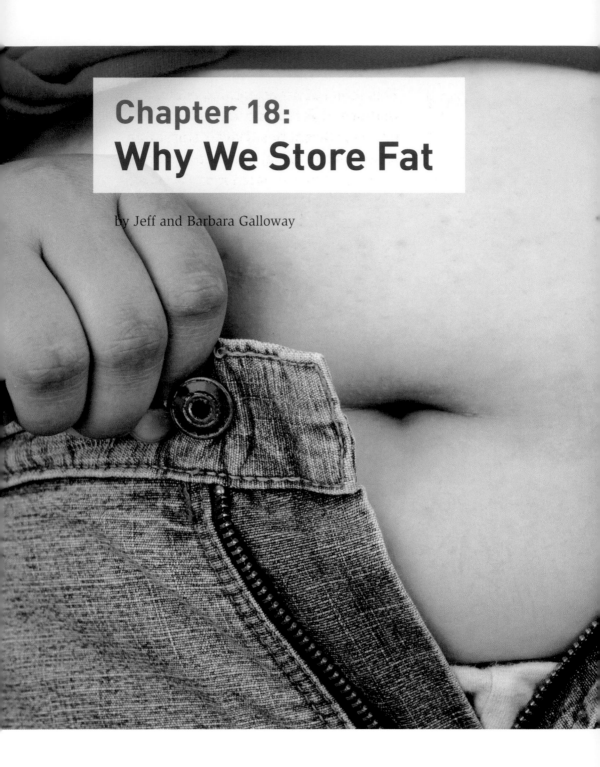

Chapter 18:
Why We Store Fat

by Jeff and Barbara Galloway

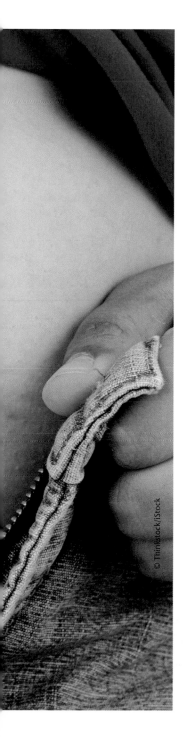

© Thinkstock/iStock

Whether we like it or not, we are hardwired with a tendency to store fat. This internal programming evolved over millions of years as a way to deal with the greatest threat to survival: starvation. Numerous internal mind-body circuits developed to promote fat storage as a hedge against famine and prolonged sickness. The ancestors who survived these repeated challenges were those with adequate fat accumulation. These genetic patterns of fat deposit govern our eating behaviors today even though food is abundantly available.

MISSION: To use your conscious brain when engaging in eating behaviors. This will be covered in chapter 19.

Simply stated, our subconscious brain (SCB), is on a mission to store fat efficiently when food is available, and hold on to body fat for use when intake is low.

- SBC circuits stimulate the desire to eat when food is available.
- Our appetite circuit is turned on when food is available and is not turned off until we have usually eaten much more than we have burned since the last meal.
- The extra volume not only promoted fat accumulation but a volume of vitamins, minerals, and protein.

- We are rewarded with a dopamine "hit" for eating sugar and fat—the most efficient nutrients for conversion into body fat.
- Subconscious dopamine reward patterns are stimulated when these junk foods are around—with no accountability as we eat and eat and eat.

Set point circuit—This denotes the amount of fat that is programmed for the individual to have in storage at various stages of life. Lowest level tends to be in the early 20s. Each year, a bit more fat is added in a vast number of storage areas throughout the body. When we put ourselves through a starvation diet and lose a lot of fat quickly, set point remembers the before-diet level. When normal eating resumes, set point triggers a hunger response, day after day, until the level has been achieved—usually with an additional amount.

Runners tend to add few pounds or no pounds if they use the conscious brain instead of the SBC to monitor eating behaviors. Countless recreational runners have told me their journey of losing 20, 50, 100, and even 150+ pounds when they got into a regular running program. Research shows that running significantly activates the conscious brain. Other research shows that when a person starts running they tend to change their diet in a positive way. You'll find a plan to use the frontal lobe for fat burning later in the chapter.

Conditions that Compromise Your Fat-Burning

Stress stimulates subconscious eating patterns—SBC, when we allow it to be in control, will monitor overall stress and will stimulate the release of negative attitude hormones when stress is too high. This stimulates an appetite for dopamine releasing foods to counter the negative attitude. Many runners justify "carbohydrate loading" by SBC snacking to counter the stress of an upcoming race or long run, for example.

So it is common, when stressed or very tired, to subconsciously reach for sugary, salty, and fatty snacks to get a dose of dopamine. Unfortunately the reward is very temporary and then requires multiple doses, with no accountability. Again, the way you can gain control is to have a conscious strategy which is listed next.

Damage from addictive eating patterns—Dr. Pam Peeke, in her book *The Hunger Fix*, has noted the research showing how addictive eating patterns can damage the natural reward centers of the brain so that more and more junk food is needed for gratification. Dr. Peeke lists healthy eating and exercise tips to restore the natural rewards.

The starvation circuit—When you wait more than about two hours between a meal or snack, your SCB senses that you're starting into a food deprivation phase. The longer you wait, the more you compromise your fat burning goals as the starvation circuit takes action:

- Triggers the release of fat-depositing enzymes. These hang around the gut and go into action when you eat again—depositing more than usual into body fat.
- Lowers your metabolism rate—the longer you wait, the lower it will go. You feel lethargic, sleepy, don't move around as much, don't feel like exercising, and don't burn many calories.
- Stimulates the memory in the appetite circuit to crave more when you start eating again.

Snacks that are too high in sugar—A simple carbohydrate snack (sugar, starch), after three to five hours of no food intake or when hungry, can trigger a dopamine reflex eating pattern. Each taste of sugar stimulates a strong craving for more and often results in a blood sugar roller coaster: boosting the blood glucose temporarily which stimulates an insulin to lower the blood sugar lower than before. You're down in the dumps again. The solution is to eat wholesome fruits, vegetables, and grains with a source of protein such as an apple with peanut butter or a handful of trail mix (nuts and dried fruit).

The Low-Carbohydrate (LC) Diet Scam

There is no doubt that low-carb diets can help you lose weight....water weight. Such a loss is superficial and easily gained back. The basic problem is that your brain's only fuel is blood glucose. Low-carb diets reduce this vital energy source, and the brain triggers the starvation circuit.

Here's how it works. To keep the brain energized you need to keep your blood sugar at a good level all day. In addition, runners need a quick energy source called glycogen, which is a basic form of carbohydrate that is stored in the muscles, liver, and other areas. It must be replenished every day. The storage areas for glycogen are limited. A good quantity of water (needed in the use of glycogen) is stored along with the glycogen.

By starving themselves of carbohydrates, low-carb (LC) dieters experience a severe reduction in glycogen—and energy level. But if the glycogen isn't there, water is not stored either. The elimination of these two substances can result in significant weight loss within days—or until the glycogen stores are depleted.

Fat levels can actually increase during a low-carb diet if a person overeats total calories. A primary ingredient in low-carb diets is fat (think salad dressing), which is directly deposited on the body if you over indulge. But dieters don't realize this because the scales are showing a total loss—due to the water/glycogen reduction. Because of low blood sugar levels, dieters tend to exercise less—so "calories in" tend to be higher than "calories burned."

The big surprise: When the low-carb diet is finished, and they replace water and glycogen later, the weight goes back on. Soon the overall body weight is greater than before because of the excess calories/lower exertion during the diet period.

Because the glycogen energy source is low or depleted, low carbers will not have much energy for exercise. This is why you will hear people on this diet complain of major fatigue, lack of desire to exercise, inability to finish a workout, and sometimes lack of mental focus (low glycogen means less fuel for the brain).

Even if you "tough it out" or cheat on the diet a little, your capacity to do even moderately strenuous exertions will be greatly reduced. With your energy stores near empty, exercising becomes a real struggle, and no fun. The reduction in exercise and movement in general usually results in burning fewer calories as you go about your life activities.

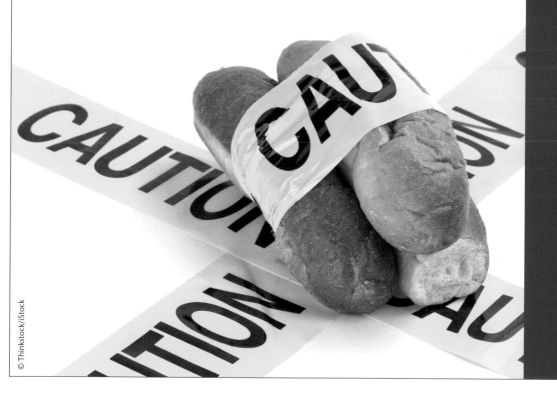

© Thinkstock/iStock

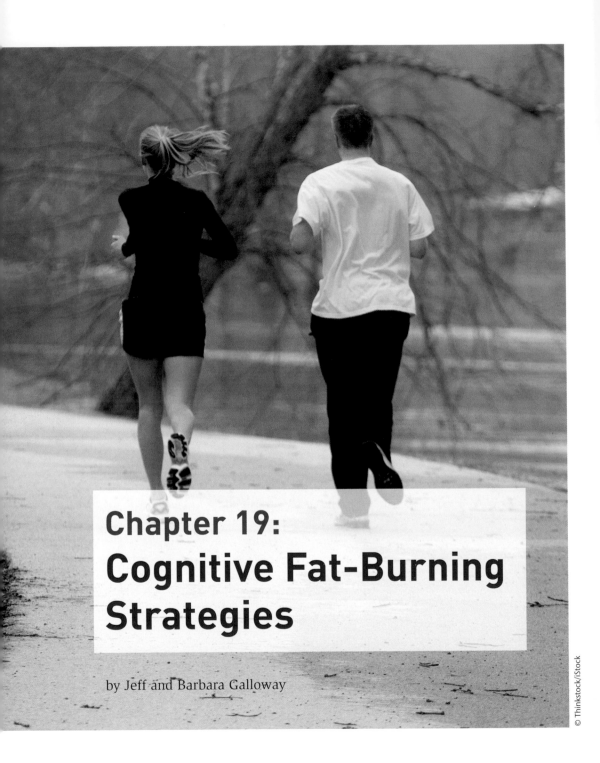

Chapter 19:
Cognitive Fat-Burning Strategies

by Jeff and Barbara Galloway

© Thinkstock/iStock

As noted in the beginning of this book, you have the power in your conscious brain to take control over your eating, to change your body and life for the better. You must activate this executive control center to stay in charge, and the tools below can help you do this. Each one connects to a cognitive strategy to keep you focused on what you are going to eat, and then account for each item consumed. This keeps you in the frontal lobe and away from subconscious brain (SCB) emotional eating.

Your mental focus will allow you to 1) control intake and 2) increase the number of gentle running and walking steps. The combination of the two has helped thousands burn 10 to 100 + pounds while feeling empowered.

> You can eat the foods you like—you just have to account for them in the budget. Gentle exercise is preferable to strenuous, painful exercise. No huffing exercises.
> Gentle exercise bestows a better attitude and mental focus—reinforcing healthy eating.

Review of Fat Accumulation

Energy production is the #1 priority in our mind–body network.
- Fat is our genetic insurance policy against energy interruption.
- We can easily add a bit more fat each year due to less activity and overeating.
- The set point maintains fat storage.
- The lowest set point is experienced in the early 20s.
- Men and women deposit fat differently.
- Restrictive diets don't work because of the "starvation reflex".
- Waiting too long to eat triggers the starvation reflex.

Managing the Calorie Budget

Buy a journal: Carry it everywhere…write down everything you eat! Go to an office supply store or a book store and find a journal format that you like, fits into your purse.

When you eat or drink anything (including water), quickly write down the food eaten before or immediately after consuming it.

At first you may need to measure items with a food scale, measuring spoons and cups. Learn portion sizes of your favorite foods. **Hint:** A *portion* is about the size of your fist, or a deck of playing cards.

When eating in restaurants: Ask for nutritional contents or recipes.

You need 10 calories per pound for basal metabolism.

Calorie budget should be increased with exercise (see the calorie burning table in this book).

Recommended daily calorie deficit: No more than 500 calories per day.

Other tools that can keep you in the conscious brain, focusing on good food choices and infusing gentle exercise into your life:

- Use a resource like this book or *Running and Fat Burning for Women* by Barbara and Jeff Galloway for back-up information and to understand the process.
- Set your calorie deficit goal each day (250 is the maximum recommended).
- Set up a calorie "budget" for each day, including foods that taste good.
- Get a step counter and increase the number of running steps and walking steps to achieve your calorie deficit (10,000+ steps).
- As you monitor your eating and exercise, you gain control and can take action to improve the efficiency of the process. You control your budget and stay in the conscious brain.

- By increasing walking steps to 10,000 (and beyond), you can eat a few more calories and still lose fat. This is accounted for as you log into the app or website.

How to modify SBC eating behaviors:
- Focus on each food choice, all day. Estimate calorie content before eating anything—this shifts consciousness to frontal lobe.
- Write down every item you eat: amount and brand.
- If there are foods that you really love, which are hazardous to your goals, eat small amounts and account for them. Prolonged deprivation of foods that you love and have eaten regularly can lead to deprivation and cravings. Reduce the amount of each snack and gradually taper down the frequency.
- Search for healthy, good tasting foods that can replace the hazard foods.
- Reward yourself for making progress with non-food items, like a timer, step counter.
- At the end of each day, do the accounting on your website or app.
- Don't just look at calorie balance—see if you were ingesting enough calcium, iron, B vitamins, etc.
- Don't panic if you were low in some areas—you can make up during the next week as you look at the totals each day.

A Burning Strategy

1. Set a realistic calorie deficit—between 50 and 250 calories per day.
By focusing on a cognitive strategy you engage the frontal lobe and assume conscious control over eating behaviors. This type of modest deficit can be sustainable, whereas higher deficits are likely to engage the starvation circuit in your brain, which has memory. While you are depriving yourself of the amount that the starvation circuit feels is adequate, the circuit remembers. When you resume eating regularly, it triggers a hunger response, resulting in overeating. This is one reason why starvation diets don't work and result in more fat deposited (than was lost) during the year after the diet is terminated.

2. **Get a step counter and strive to take 10,000 steps or more per day.**
    Walking steps, taken in amounts of 100 to 1,000 increments at various times of the day, burn fat, increase your calorie budget for the day, and don't tend to trigger the hunger circuit. Many runners find that increasing walking steps creates most or all of the calorie deficit they need, requiring little or no change in food intake or running mileage increase to produce the calorie burn desired.

3. **Write down everything you eat.**
    This is the most powerful tool to control food intake. The act of writing, by itself, activates the conscious brain, triggering circuits that monitor food intake, avoid decadent food, and allow you to stay away from subconscious gratification eating.

4. **Each day, account for your nutrients.**
    Use the app or website of your choice and see if your diet gave you the vitamins, minerals, protein, and other nutrients needed. This conscious brain exercise will allow you to search for and prepare foods that fill in the deficits. You'll also receive your calorie balance for the day. By mentally focusing on this at least once a day, you'll tend to make executive decisions about what to eat instead of slipping into subconscious gratification eating patterns. There are many free websites such as www.fitday.com and www.supertracker.usda.gov with tools to help you in calorie accounting, charting progress, and searching for foods.

5. Run/walk for a minimum of 60 minutes on the two maintenance days and 90 minutes on the non-long-run weekend. Avoid huffing and puffing and choose a gentle pace that you can sustain. Fast running will leave you exhausted. Use the run-walk-run strategy that works best for you, but don't be shy about using more walk breaks if you are huffing and puffing or are not feeling as good as usual, especially during the first 15 minutes of the run. The fat-burning circuits don't reach their maximum capacity until about 40 minutes into the run. Continuing to run at that point extends and maintains fat-burning adaptations. If you're not running 60 or 90 minutes now, gradually work up to that level.

6. Ensure that your blood sugar level (BSL) is adequate during the half hour before a workout or race. When you're in a calorie deficit, you're more likely to have a drop in the BSL at various times of the day—especially in the afternoon. By eating a blood sugar booster snack you will tend to feel more motivated to start the run, and feel better during the run. On early morning runs, the BSL is usually adequate if you ate sufficiently the day and evening before. If you did not eat adequately the day before and need a before-workout snack, consume it within 30 minutes before the start of your run, with a 2-4 oz of water.

7. Eat a reloading snack, preferably within 30 minutes of finishing a workout or back your run into a meal. (See caloric recommendations later in this chapter, based upon distance run.) This will curb your appetite and help you control your appetite.

The Burning Zone

Avoid a radical change—Every year I hear from several dozen runners who have to abandon a training program because of dietary issues. They started or re-started their running career and made a radical change in their diets at the same time. After several weeks or months they either felt chronically fatigued, or experienced some digestive issues. A more successful strategy is to make small and gradual changes, while monitoring nutrition using a website such as www.fitday.com or www.supertracker.usda.gov.

Gentle exercise is important—To lose weight you must create a calorie deficit. You can contribute to this deficit by monitoring food intake and by exercising at an aerobic level—gentle exertion so that the muscles can easily get the oxygen they need to burn fat. If you run too fast, oxygen needs increase dramatically and cannot be supplied by the blood stream. In this case, the brain shifts out of the fat-burning zone and burns glycogen—the stored form of carbohydrate.

Time goals? It's not a good idea to try to lose fat while training for a time goal because of the anaerobic speed workouts needed to run faster. Fast running uses more glycogen and can result in a hunger response, usually in the evening or the day after a strenuous fast run. Reloading with a proper recovery meal can help reduce this hunger reflex, but may not eliminate it.

Again, it's also not a good idea to change diet dramatically when training for a challenging goal. Many runners think they are improving diet by cutting out a lot of foods they believe are "fattening." This often results in not getting adequate vitamins, minerals, or protein and lowers performance potential.

Running Can Be a Catalyst

At every big event expo, I talk to at least a dozen runners who tell me that they lost 30-150 + pounds or more because they set the goal of finishing a 10K, half marathon, or marathon. In some cases it took 10 years, but as I talked with each there were two concepts that were shared and followed:

1. They set up a cognitive plan to monitor eating. This empowers the conscious brain to choose and account for food consumed. This frontal lobe brain component overrides the subconscious brain, which can stimulate subconscious gratification snacks (Suddenly you realize that the potato chip bag is empty and you are the only one who has been eating them.)
2. They used one of my training books and kept up with the training schedule. Exercise does a lot more than just burn calories. When you run or walk, for more than about 30 minutes, you activate circuits in the brain that burn fat, control appetite, and make you feel good about what you are doing. This reduces the chance that the subconscious brain will trigger gratification eating to combat the blues.

Curbing Hunger

Eat a reloading snack preferably within 30 minutes of finishing a run, easily done by backing your run into a meal. Circuits in the brain are triggered to reload the fuel burned during the first 30 minutes of your run. This is when your muscles are more receptive to replacing depleted muscle glygogen stores. If you don't reload within 30 minutes of finishing, you may not have the ideal quantity of muscle fuel during the first part of your next run, if you are doing double workouts and will be training again within six to eight hours.

Many runners tell me that avoiding the reloading meal leaves them more hungry later in the day—or the next day. The best mix of reloading nutrients, according to research, is four times more carbs than protein. The brain's hunger/satisfaction circuit is more likely to be on the satisfaction side if you have consumed your snack within the half hour after completion.

Jeff's Guidelines for the reloading Snack
- 4 miles or less—100 calories
- 4-8 miles—150 calories
- 8-12 miles—200 calories
- 12-14 miles—250 calories
- 14 + miles—300 calories

How to Reduce Hunger

1. Exercise in the morning. Morning workouts will get your healthy habits started on the right foot.
2. Drink 8 oz of water with every snack or meal.
3. Eat more often and smaller portions. If you usually eat a chicken breast, salad, or a piece of bread with peanut butter, every 3-4 hours, eat one-third to one-half of either every 2-2.5 hours, with 6-8 oz of water.
4. Strive for wholesome fruits, vegetables, and grains in your snacks with an accompaniment of protein. This can leave you feeling satisfied longer. See the next section for more information.

5. If you dearly love a certain sugar snack, eat a small amount to get a taste after a meal that has some protein and fat—and account for it in your calorie budget for the day.

6. Don't eat a sugar snack by itself when you are hungry.

Key Fat-Burning Principles

Eating every 2-3 hours may help you lose 8-10 pounds a year—If you are hungry but have not eaten for about three hours, your body senses that it is going into a starvation mode, and slows down the metabolism rate, while increasing the production of fat-depositing enzymes. This means that you will be lethargic and will not burn as many calories as is normal and that you probably won't be as mentally and physically alert as you could be.

Burn more fat by eating more often—What a deal! If the starvation reflex starts working after three hours, then think about eating every two hours. A person who now eats two to three times a day might lose more extra pounds a year when he or she shifts to eating six to nine times a day. This assumes equal calories are eaten under each meal frequency pattern.

Big meals slow you down—Big meals are a big production for the digestive system. Blood is diverted to the long and winding intestine and the stomach. Because of the workload, the body tends to reduce blood flow to other areas, leaving you feeling more lethargic.

Small meals speed you up—Smaller amounts of food can usually be processed quickly without putting a burden on the digestive system.

Eating frequently helps you manage the set point—When you wait more than three hours between meals, the set point engages the starvation reflex. But if you eat every two to three hours, the starvation reflex is often not engaged—due to the regular supply of food.

Motivation increases when you eat more often—Low motivation in the afternoon is often due to not eating regularly enough during the day: not eating breakfast, not eating enough total calories, and eating very little from lunch until afternoon workout time. If you have not eaten for four hours or more, and you're scheduled for a workout that afternoon, you will often not feel very motivated because of low blood sugar and lethargy. You can turn this around, even when you've had a bad eating day, by having a snack 30 minutes before exercise. A fibrous energy bar with a cup of coffee (tea, diet drink) can reverse the negative mindset and energy deficit. Eating breakfast and then eating every two to three hours can keep your energy flowing.

Satisfaction From a Small Meal—To Avoid Overeating

The number of calories you eat per day can be reduced by choosing foods and combinations of foods that leave you satisfied longer. Best choices are protein-rich foods and high-fiber foods. For some people, sugar can be a problem in terms of calorie control and satisfaction. When you drink a beverage with sugar in it, the sugar will be processed very quickly, and some will be hungry within 30 minutes—even after consuming a high quantity of calories. This will usually lead to three undesirable outcomes:

1. Eating more food to satisfy hunger.
2. Staying hungry and triggering the starvation reflex.
3. The extra calories are processed into fat.

Your mission is to find the right combination of foods in your small meals that will leave you satisfied for two to three hours. Then, eat another snack that will do the same. You will find a growing number of food combinations that probably have fewer calories but keep you from getting hungry until your next snack. Some popular choices include banana with peanut butter, Greek yogurt with berries, and crackers with reduced fat cheese.

Nutrients That Leave You Satisfied Longer:

Fat

A certain amount of fat in a snack or meal will leave you satisfied longer because it slows down digestion, but a little goes a long way. Excess calories of fat are easily fattening.

Bad Fat: There are two kinds of fat that have been found to cause narrowing of the arteries around the heart and leading to your brain: saturated fat and trans fat. In contrast, mono—and unsaturated fats, from vegetable sources, are often healthy—olive oil, nuts, avocado, canola oil, and safflower oil. Some fish oils have omega-3 fatty acids which have been shown to have a protective effect on the heart. Check food composition websites for this information. Most of the fat in animal products is saturated fat.

Look carefully at the labels because some prepared foods have vegetable oils that have been processed into trans fat. A wide range of baked goods and other foods have used trans fat. It helps to check the labels, and check the website or call the 800 number to ask about foods that don't break down the fat composition. Another simple solution is to simply avoid the foods that aren't well labeled—especially baked goods.

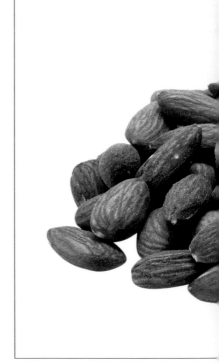

Protein—Go for the lean!

You need protein every day for rebuilding the muscle that is broken down during exercise, as well as normal wear and tear. But endurance exercisers (even runners who log high mileage) don't need to eat significantly more protein than sedentary people. But if endurance exercisers don't get adequate protein, they'll feel more aches and pains (and general weakness) sooner than average low-calorie-burning people.

Having protein with each meal will leave you feeling satisfied for a longer period of time. But eating more protein calories than you need will produce a conversion of the excess into fat. A general guideline for daily intake of protein is one-half a gram for every pound of bodyweight or about 1 g of protein for each kg of bodyweight).

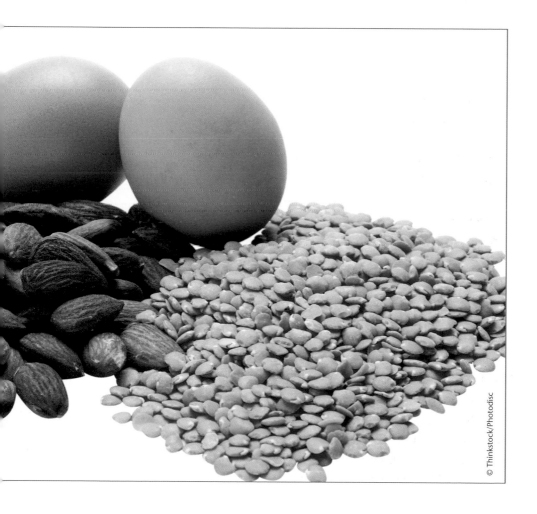

© Thinkstock/Photodisc

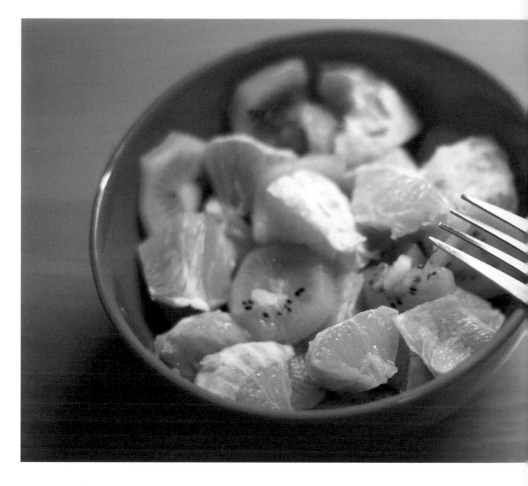

Complex carbohydrates give you a "discount" and a "grace period."
Foods such as celery, beans, cabbage, spinach, turnip greens, grape nuts, whole-grain cereal can burn up to more calories in digestion. After dinner, for example, you have the opportunity to burn off any excess calories that you acquired during the day with walking around the neighborhood. The extra fiber in these foods leaves you satisfied longer.

Fat + Protein + Complex Carbs = SATISFACTION
Eating a snack that has a variety of these three satisfaction ingredients, will lengthen the time that you'll feeling satisfied—even after small meals. These three items take longer to digest, and therefore keep you feel fuller for longer.

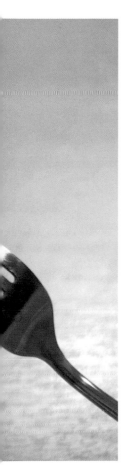

Other Important Nutrients...

Fiber

When fiber is put into foods, it slows down digestion and maintains the feeling of satisfaction longer. Soluble fiber, such as oat bran, seems to bestow a longer feeling of satisfaction than unsoluble fiber such as wheat bran. But any type of fiber will help in this regard.

Some carbohydrates can be easily overconsumed and stored as body fat. These are the feel-good foods: candy, baked sweets, starches like mashed potatoes and rice, sugar drinks (including fruit juice and sports drinks), and most desserts. Some simple carb snacks can speed reloading when consumed within 30 minutes after finishing a strenuous workout. But when you're on a fat-burning mission, you need to minimize the amount of calories you consume. Again, this is simply a matter of budgeting.

Foods filled with refined sugar can be quickly digested so that you get little or no lasting satisfaction from them. They may leave you craving more of them, which, if denied, can activate a starvation reflex. Because they are processed quickly, you become hungry relatively quickly and will tend to eat more, accumulating extra calories that can easily end up as fat at the end of the day.

As mentioned in the last chapter, it is never a good idea to eliminate all of the simple carb foods that you like. The worst situation is to say "I'll never eat another...". This starts the ticking of a starvation-reflex time bomb: At some point in the future, when the food is around and no one else is, you will eat and eat. Keep taking a bite or two of the foods you dearly love when you have cravings—but only a bite or two. At the same time, cultivate an appreciation for the taste of foods with more fiber and little or no refined sugar (and a reduced amount of fat).

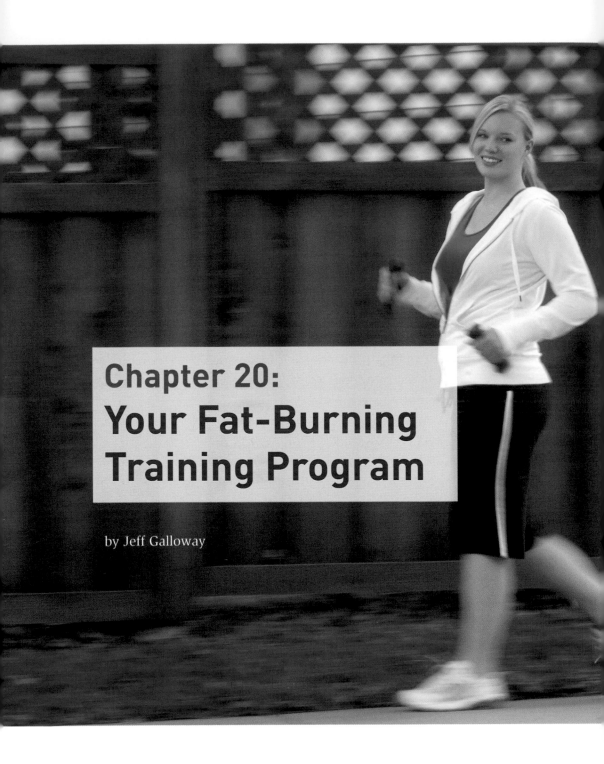

Chapter 20:
Your Fat-Burning Training Program

by Jeff Galloway

Gentle-paced running can allow tens of thousands of leg muscle cells to adapt to fat-burning and significantly increase your calorie-burning capacity so that you can run longer before you run out of muscle glycogen and "hit the wall." Just as important, running activates brain circuits that help you focus on food intake. I've spoken to thousands who tried many ways to lose weight and it came back on—until they started running and eating better.

Concepts of Fat-Burning

- Aerobic, easy running burns fat. This means no huffing and puffing. This does not automatically mean that you will lose body fat. You need to create a calorie deficit to do that.
- Liberal walk breaks help you stay aerobic—chapter 21 for more on the run-walk-run method.
- Long, aerobic runs can adapt the muscle cells to be better fat burners so they have greater endurance. The longer your run, the more calories you can burn.
- During speed training and fast running you're not burning fat, but glycogen (stored form of carbohydrate). When you burn glycogen, and don't reload within 30-60 minutes, the hunger circuit is triggered.
- Walking is aerobic—the more steps you take, the more calories you burn.
- Monitor food intake and exercise by using one of the programs or websites.
- Gentle cross-training will increase calorie burning, either on non-running days or as a second workout on a running day.

Exercise + Mental Focus = Fat Management

- Exercise is your furnace that burns calories all day—and can help you lose fat and keep it off.
- When running is gentle and balanced, you turn on circuits to feel better during and after.
- The run-walk-run method can keep you in a sustainable exercise mode.
- Aches and pains from running are self-induced and can be virtually eliminated.
- Exercising too hard or too long (for you on that day) will often trigger an appetite increase.
- Shorter segments of running and walking, can burn calories without the appetite increase.
- Your calorie burning starts each day with a single step—and each step afterward burns more calories.
- Exercise extends length and quality of life—enjoy your grandchildren with good health.

It's a fact that running can lower blood pressure, help you manage cholesterol, reduce your chance of cancer, stroke, and heart disease, as it extends your lifespan with quality. The best benefits as identified by research are the enhancements to the brain circuits that are turned on by each run: a better attitude, more vitality, personal empowerment. The only time each day when I feel totally in control over my attitude is during my run, and this positive effect lingers afterward.

It is also clear that you can lose weight efficiently through running. Each month I hear from dozens of former obese people who tried dozens of diets and quick weight-loss programs with no success. But after running and focusing on food, they shed 30, 50, even 100 + pounds and kept it off.

Thousands of runners have told me that they couldn't lose that last 10 or 20 pounds by running alone. But when they applied the principles of eating with a purpose in this book, they not only burned it off—they kept it off.

YOU CAN DO THIS TOO!

Gentle exercise builds self-respect, personal empowerment, and the will to make changes in your life. If you will simply get out and move your feet to get your steps or do your run-walk-run, the body works better as the brain focuses better. Yes, during and after each workout you make yourself more attractive, more energized, more productive, and more relaxed because you spent the mental and physical energy to run.

Even a gentle run for a few minutes makes you feel better than before. You discover or rediscover simple, life-enhancing sensations:
- That you can get out the door on a busy day and get things done afterward
- That you can keep going when you didn't think you could
- That you solve problems (personal, job, family) during and after a workout
- That you are more productive after a gentle workout, with more energy to do things
- That you think more clearly when you've exercised at a conservative effort level

If exercise hurts, you've been running too hard, there is something wrong with your orthopedic condition, or you are not doing the workout correctly, for you. The program in this book will make you the captain of your running ship. Once you feel the continuing stream of benefits, you will look forward to the next run.

Health benefits without weight loss—Even if there is not a weight loss, regular exercise delivers a series of significant health benefits. Studies at the Cooper Clinic, founded by Dr. Kenneth Cooper in Dallas TX, and other organizations, have shown that even obese people lower their risk factors for heart disease and cancer when they exercise regularly. They also feel better about themselves and accomplish more when regularly exercising.

Exercise does not have to hurt—And should make you feel better. Gentle exertion triggers brain circuits that rev up your metabolism so that you feel more energized during the day. The positive attitude effects of gentle exercise leave you feeling better than before you started—and the boost can last for hours.

Aerobic Exercise Burns Calories—No Huffing and Puffing
- There must be enough oxygen delivered by the blood during exercise for you to exercise with enjoyment
- When walking or doing any gentle exercise that does not stress the muscles, the normal flow of blood will deliver enough oxygen to burn calories.
- If you're not huffing and puffing, you're in the aerobic or fat-burning zone, but this does not mean you will lose body fat. Losing fat requires a calorie deficit for the day.
- But when you work out too hard for you on that day, and you can't carry on a conversation, the muscles are working beyond their current limit. You're not having much fun.
- The muscles will then shift to glycogen for energy, leaving a lot of waste (lactic acid).
- As your legs fill up with this residue, they get tighter, performance drops, and exercise is no fun—muscles hurt.
- Hard exercise reduces motivation. Your subconscious brain monitors stress and also keeps track of the available supply of blood glucose, the fuel source for the brain. As the stress level goes up and the glucose supply goes down during a hard workout, the subconscious brain (SBC) triggers a number of negative hormones sending negative messages such as "it isn't your day" or "this is boring" or "why are you doing this" to preserve its fuel source.

You're training the muscle cells to run longer and this can help you lose weight—Exercising at an easy effort will tend to keep you in the aerobic zone, minute by minute, hour by hour. Very gentle exercise done regularly (even in short segments) will make you fit enough to gradually increase the length of one longer workout a week. As this long one increases, you will transform thousands of muscle cells into calorie burners.

You have two types of fuel on board: glycogen and fat—Glycogen is the stored form of carbohydrate and is the ready-reserve fuel supply for the brain and muscles. It can be used from the beginning of any run as a primary fuel. But if you exercise too hard, waste products such as lactic acid build up quickly, making it difficult to continue running. Burning glycogen, the brain's reserve fuel, can trigger a hunger response during the next 36 hours. The supply of glycogen is limited in the human body and must be replenished or you won't have adequate fuel at the beginning of your next run.

Exercise Is Fun—A Fat-Burning Program That Can Be Inserted Into Life

- One gentle long workout a week, gradually building up to 90 + min
- Two gentle 60-min runs
- Two to three optional weekly cross-training exercise sessions or gentle walks of 45 + min (exercise that you enjoy)
- Walking 10,000 steps a day in your daily activities minimum (walking and running)
- No huffing and puffing on any run
- See chapter 21 for running and walking strategies

Runner Eating Myths

I'll lose a lot of weight when training for a 10K, half marathon or marathon— In fact, losing a lot of weight the wrong way can leave you weak, without the energy or essential nutrients needed for endurance performance. Too much of a calorie deficit can result in low blood sugar with inadequate mental or physical energy for finishing a run—or even starting one.

One can eat anything desired when training for a distance event, this myth is more of an excuse that runners give themselves for gratification eating. Because they finished a 12-mile training run, some runners give themselves permission to eat a box of Girl Scout cookies or to eat big meals for three days afterward. To avoid this, you must stay focused on your calorie budget and account for everything you eat.

Beginner (just started or just started again)

WEEK#	TUE	THU	WEEKEND
1	10 min	13 min	15 min
2	15 min	8 min	18 min
3	20 min	23 min	23 min
4	25 min	28 min	33 min
5	30 min	33 min	43 min
6	35 min	38 min	50 min
7	40 min	43 min	60 min
8	45 min	48 min	45 min
9	50 min	53 min	70 min
10	55 min	58 min	50 min
11	60 min	60 min	80 min
12	60 min	60 min	55 min
13	60 min	60 min	90 min
14	60 min	60 min	60 min
15	60 min	60 min	90 min

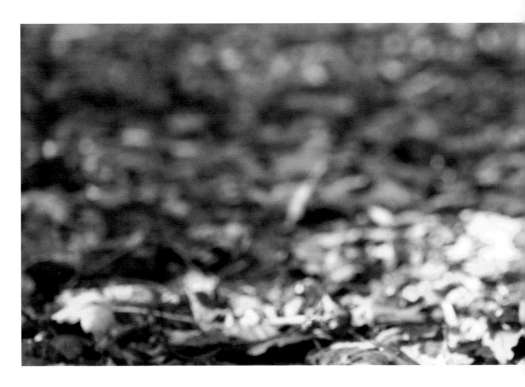

Veteran Runner (running 3 days a week for at least a year)

WEEK#	TUE	THU	WEEKEND
1	30 min	30 min	45 min
2	35 min	35 min	50 min
3	40 min	40 min	60 min
4	45 min	45 min	45 min
5	50 min	50 min	70 min
6	55 min	55 min	50 min
7	60 min	60 min	70 min
8	60 min	60 min	60 min
9	60 min	60 min	80 min
10	60 min	60 min	70 min
11	60 min	60 min	90 min
12	60 min	60 min	80 min
13	60 min	60 min	90 min
14	60 min	60 min	80 min
15	60 min	60 min	90 min

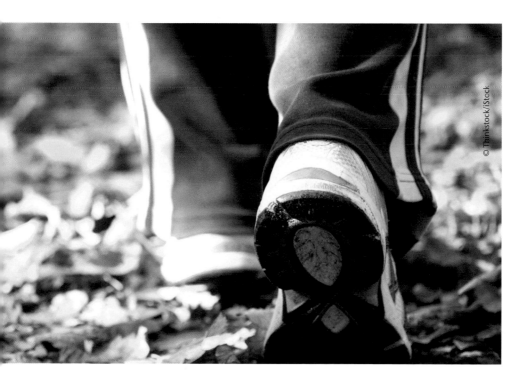

© Thinkstock/iStock

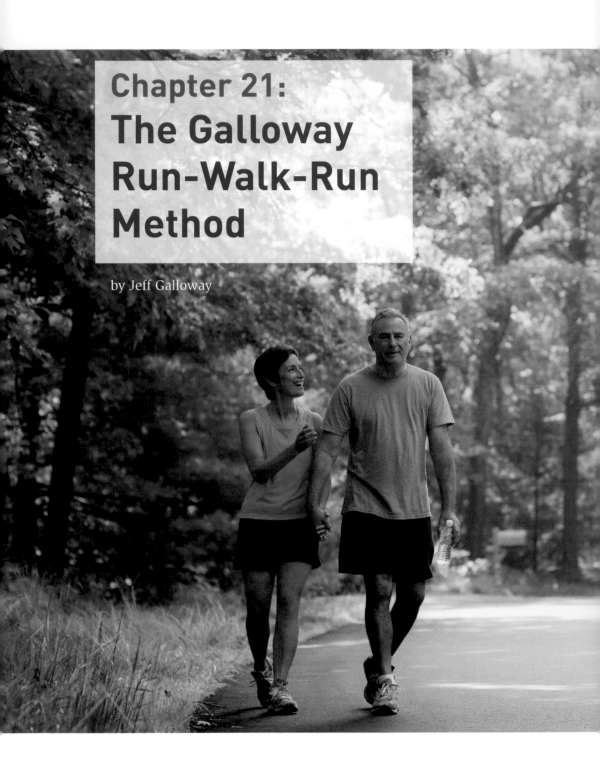

Chapter 21: The Galloway Run-Walk-Run Method

by Jeff Galloway

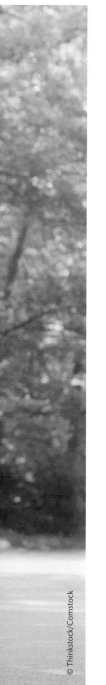

The scheduled use of walk breaks, can keep you in the fat-burning zone, while allowing you to gain control over fatigue.

I believe that most runners want to be in control over how they feel during a workout. The simple insertion of walk breaks, can allow each runner to adjust the effort level which is so important for enjoying exercise. If you are exercising at a gentle level, you can exercise longer and burn more calories.

But if you keep pushing the effort during a workout, at some point, the muscles can't get the oxygen needed to burn fat. As the fuel supply shifts to glycogen (stored carbohydrate), you will acquire an "oxygen debt" signified by huffing and puffing. This makes fat-burning impossible and running more difficult and less enjoyable.

By keeping the exertion level low enough, the muscles can pull oxygen from the arterial blood constantly pumping through. Walk breaks can not only keep the exertion level at aerobic levels, they allow the running muscles to maintain stamina and endurance.

Walk breaks act as a shock absorber to the exertion system. The proven strategy of run-walk-run gives you control over how you feel and how strong you will be throughout the workout (especially at the end). As you adjust the frequency or duration of the walk breaks you become the captain of your running ship.

Strategic walk breaks allow people citizens to ease into running and finish half or full marathons in six to nine months. Surprisingly, they allow veteran runners to run faster, stay injury free, and enjoy running more. Here's how it works.

© Thinkstock/Comstock

Walk Before You Get Tired

Most of us, even when untrained, can walk for several miles before fatigue sets in, because walking is an activity that we are bio-engineered to do for hours. Running is more work, because you have to lift your body off the ground and then absorb the shock of the landing, over and over. This is why the continuous use of the running muscles will produce fatigue, aches, and pains much more quickly.

Running also uses fuel much more quickly than walking. The longer you run non-stop, the more likely you will move out of the aerobic, fat-burning zone, and into the glycogen-burning zone. If you insert a walk break into a run before your running muscles start to get tired, you allow the muscles to recover instantly—increasing your capacity for exercise. With each walk break you extend your time in the aerobic zone.

The Huff and Puff Rule
If you are breathing so hard that you cannot carry on a continuous conversation or sing a song, you are working too hard. Take more frequent walk breaks or shorten running segments or both.

The method part involves having a strategy. By focusing on doable amounts of running with enough walking to erase the fatigue, you will gain control over your fat-burning. Using this fatigue-reduction tool early will also save muscle resources and bestow the mental confidence to cope with any challenges that may come later. Even when you don't need the extra muscle strength and resiliency bestowed by the method, you will feel better during and after your run, and finish knowing that you could have gone further. You'll be in the fat-burning zone the whole time.

Beginners: How to Use Walk Breaks

Walk only the first week or so. When a 30-minute walk is comfortable, insert short segments of running, into each minute of your walk. This allows your muscles to gradually adapt to running, without getting overwhelmed. Over the next four to six weeks you can gradually add a few more seconds of running, subtracting seconds of walking as feels comfortable. But be prepared to drop back to more walking if you're not feeling good on a given day. For more information, with a six-month beginner program, see my book *Running: Getting Started*.

1. Start by running for 5-10 seconds and walking 1-2 minutes.
2. If you feel good during and after the run, continue with this ratio. If not, run less until you feel good.
3. After three to six sessions at the ratio, add 5-10 seconds of running, maintaining the same amount of walking.
4. When you can run for 30 seconds, gradually reduce the walking time to 30 seconds every three to six sessions.
5. When 30 seconds/30 seconds feels too easy, gradually increase the running time, 5-10 sec every three to six sessions.
6. On any given day, when you need more walking, do it. Don't ever be afraid to drop back to make the run more fun and less tiring.

Veterans: Walk breaks allow you to take control over fatigue, in advance while maximizing fat-burning. You can not only enjoy every run—you'll probably run faster in races. Surprisingly, when non-stop marathoners use the right run-walk-run strategy, the average time improvement is 13 minutes. By taking walk breaks early and often you can feel strong, even after a run that is very long for you. Even elite runners find that walk breaks on long runs allow them to recover faster. There is no need to reach the end of a run feeling exhausted—if you insert enough walk breaks, for you, on that day.

Run-Walk-Run Strategies for Veterans

PACE PER MILE	STRATEGY
8 min/mi	Run 4 min/walk 30 sec or run 2 min/walk 15 sec
9 min/mi	Run 4 min/walk 1 min or run 2 min/walk 30 sec or run 60/walk 15
10 min/mi	Run 3 min/walk 1 min or run 90 sec/walk 30 sec or run 60 sec/walk 20 sec
11 and 12 min/mi	Run 2 min/walk 1 min or run 60 sec/walk 30 sec or 40/20 or 30/15
13 and 14 min/mi	Run 1 min/walk 1 min or 30/30 or 20/20 or 15/15 or 10/10
15 and 16 min/mi	Run 10 min/walk 20 or Run 15/walk 30 or 20/40
17 and 18 min/mi	Run 10/walk 30 or run 15/walk 45 or run 20/walk 60
19 and 20 min/mi	Run 5 sec/walk 20 or run 10 sec/walk 40 or run 12/walk 48 or run 15/walk 60

Walk breaks....

- Give you control over your level of fatigue.
- Keep you in the fat-burning zone.
- Erase fatigue.
- Push back your tiredness "wall".
- Allow for endorphins to collect during each walk break—you feel good!
- Break up the distance into manageable units. ("one more minute until a walk break").
- Speed recovery.
- Reduce the chance of aches, pains, and injury.
- Allow you to feel good afterward—doing what you need to do without debilitating fatigue.
- Give you all of the endurance of the distance of each session—without the pain.
- Allow older or heavier runners to recover fast, and feel as good or better than other runners.

A Short and Gentle Walking Stride

It's better to walk slowly, with a short stride. There has been some irritation of the shins, when runners or walkers maintain a stride that is too long.

No Need to Ever Eliminate Walk Breaks

Some beginners assume that they must work toward the day when they don't have to take any walk breaks at all. This is up to the individual, but it is not recommended. Remember that you decide what ratio of run-walk-run to use. There is no rule that requires you to run any ratio of run-walk on any given day. I suggest that you adjust the ratio to how you feel.

How Keep Track of the Walk Breaks

There is a run-walk-run timer that beeps or vibrates to signal walk breaks. Check our website (www.jeffgalloway.com) for more information.

I've run for over 50 years and enjoy running more than ever because of walk breaks. Each run I take energizes my day. I would not be able to run almost every day if I didn't insert the walk breaks early and often. I start most runs taking a short walk break every 20-30 seconds.

Chapter 22:
Nutrition and Exercise Myths

by Nancy Clark, RD

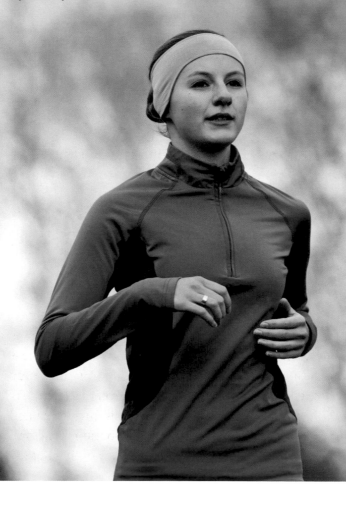

Myth: You must exercise in order to lose body fat.

To lose body fat, you must create a calorie deficit. You can create that deficit by adding exercise (which improves your overall health and fitness) or by eating fewer calories. Sick people commonly lose body fat but they do not exercise; they create a calorie deficit. Similarly, injured athletes can also lose fat despite lack of exercise. But the more common story is the following. "I gained weight when I was injured because I couldn't exercise" could more correctly be stated "I gained weight when I was injured because I was bored and depressed. I overate for comfort and entertainment."

Myth: The more you exercise, the more fat you lose.

Often, the more you exercise, the hungrier you get and—
- the more you eat, or
- the more your believe you "deserve" to eat, or
- the more you want to eat as a reward for having both gotten to the gym and survived the exercise session.

But if you spend 60 minutes in a spin class and burn off 600 calories, only to reward yourself with 12 Oreos (600 calories), you quickly wipe out your weight loss efforts in less than 3 minutes.

The effects of exercise on weight loss are complex and unclear. We know among older people (56-78 years) who participated in a vigorous walking program, daily calorie needs remained about the same (2,400 without exercise, 2,480 with exercise). How could that be? Well, the participants napped more and were 62 % less active throughout the rest of their day. (1) Another study with post-menopausal women found the same results from eight weeks of moderate exercise training. Their 24-hour energy expenditure remained similar from the start to the end of the program. (2) The bottom line: You have to eat according to your whole day's activity level, not according to how hard your trained that day.

Myth:
If you train for a marathon, your body fat will melt away.

Wishful thinking. I commonly hear marathoners, triathletes, and other highly competitive endurance athletes complain "For all the exercise I do, I should be pencil thin." They fail to lose fat because, like the fitness exercisers just described, they put all of their energy into exercising, but then tend to be quite sedentary the rest of the day as they recover from their tough workouts. A study with male endurance athletes who report a seemingly low calorie intake found they did less spontaneous activity than their peers in the non-exercise parts of their day. (3) The bottom line: You need to keep taking the stairs instead of the elevators, no matter how much you train!

Alternatively, athletes who complain they eat like a bird but fail to lose body fat may simply be under-reporting their food intake. A survey of female marathoners indicated the fatter runners under-report their food intake more so than their leaner peers. (4) Remember: Calories mindlessly eaten standing up or on-the-run count just as much as calories from meals.

Myth:
Couples who exercise together, lose fat together.

In a 16-month study looking at exercise for weight loss, men and women completed an identical amount of exercise. The men lost 11.5 pounds; the women maintained weight! (5) In another study with previously sedentary, normal weight men and women who participated in an 18-month marathon training program, the men increased their calorie intake by about 500 per day; the women increased by only 60 calories—despite having added on 50 miles per week of running. The men lost about five pounds of fat; the women two pounds. (6)

What's going on here??? Well, a husband who adds on exercise is likely to lose more weight than his wife because he's likely heftier and thereby burns more calories during the same workout. But, speaking in terms of evolution, Nature seems protective of women's role as child bearer, and wants women to maintain adequate body fat for nourishing healthy babies. Hence, women are more energy efficient. Obesity researchers at NY's Columbia University suggest a pound of weight loss in men equates to a deficit of about 2,500 calories, while women need a 3,500 calorie deficit!!! (7) No wonder women have a tougher time losing weight then do men....

The Bottom Line

If you are exercising to lose weight, I encourage you to separate exercise and weight. Yes, you should exercise for health, fitness, stress relief, and, most importantly, for enjoyment. (After all, the E in exercise stands for enjoyment!) I discourage you from exercising to burn off calories; that makes exercise feels like punishment for having excess body fat. When exercise is something you do to your body, rather than do for your body, you'll eventually quit exercising. Bad idea. Pay attention to your calorie intake. Knocking off just 100 calories a day from your evening snacks can theoretically result in 10 pounds a year of fat loss. Seems simpler than hours of sweating...?

References:

1. Goran, Am J Physiol 263:E950, 1992
2. Keytel, Int J Sport Nutr 11:226, 2001
3. Thompson, Med Sci Sports Exerc 27::347, 1995
4. Edwards, Med Sci Sports Exer 25:1398, 1993
5. Donnelly, Arch Intern Med 163:1343, 2003
6. Janssen, Int J Sports Med, 10:S1,1989
7. Pietrobelli Int J Obes Relat Metab Disord 26:1339, 2002

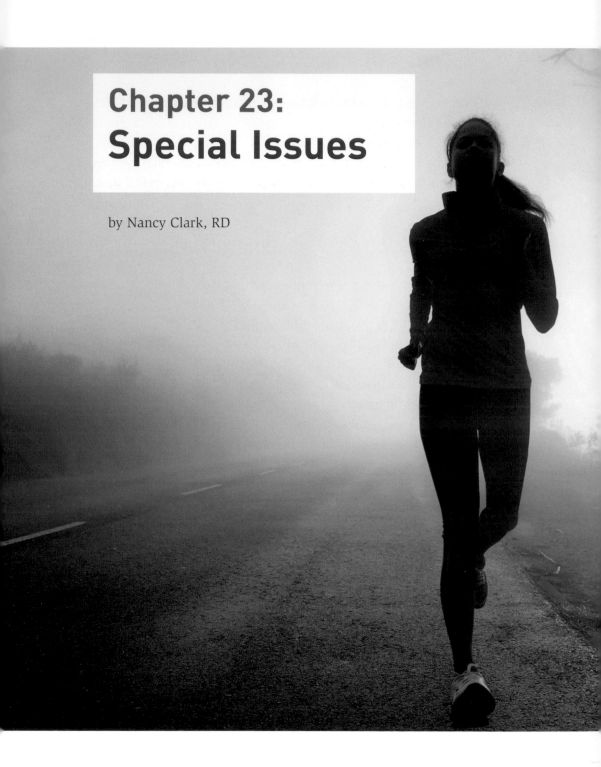

Chapter 23:
Special Issues

by Nancy Clark, RD

Nancy Clark on Amenorrhea

The negative aspects of amenorrhea, as reported by Nancy Clark, are the following.

- loss of calcium from the bones
- an incidence of stress fractures three times greater than average (24% of athletes with no or irregular periods experience stress fractures as compared to only 9% of regularly menstruating athletes)
- long-term problems with osteoporosis starting at an early age.
- temporary loss of the ability to conceive a child—and often difficulty getting pregnant in the future.

Amenorrhea and anorexia—Although amenorrhea exists among women with no eating disorders, loss of menses is certainly symptomatic of restrictive, anorectic-type eating behaviors. Anorexia is associated with weight loss 15% below normal for body type, intense fear of gaining weight or becoming fat, and distorted body image (i.e., claiming to feel fat even when emaciated), all of which are concerns common to female athletes. If you feel as though you or someone you know is struggling to balance food and exercise, you might want to seek counseling from a trusted physician, dietitian, or counselor. To find a local sports nutritionist, visit www.SCANdpg.org and use the referral network.

Note: Be sure to read Overcoming an Eating Disorder in chapter 26.

Suggestions for Amenorrhea

- Exercise a little bit less. Add a rest day or run fewer miles.
- Increase your eating so that your body has enough fuel to function normally. This will not make you fat and often brings back the regularity of periods.
- Eat adequate protein and calories. Amenorrheic athletes tend to eat less protein and calories than their regularly

menstruating counterparts. Even if you are a vegetarian, remember that you still need adequate protein. Eat additional calories from yogurt, fish, beans, tofu, and nuts.

- Eat at least 20% of your calories from fat. If you believe you will get fat if you eat fat, think again. Although excess calories from fat are easily fattening, some fat (20-30% of total calories; 40-60+ grams fat/day) is an appropriate part of a healthy sports diet. Nuts, peanut butter, salmon, and olive oil are healthful choices.

- If your diet allows, include small portions of red meat two to three times per week. Surveys suggest runners with amenorrhea tend to eat less red meat and are more likely to follow a vegetarian diet than their regularly menstruating counterparts. Even in the general population, vegetarian women are five times more likely to have menstrual problems than meat eaters. It's unclear why meat seems to have a protective effect upon menses.

- Maintain a calcium-rich diet to help maintain bone density. A safe target is the equivalent of three to four servings per day of low-fat milk, yogurt, and other calcium-rich foods. Being athletic, your bones benefit from the protective effect of exercise, but this does not compensate for lack of calcium nor lack of estrogen.

- Stay in touch with your OB-GYN. Amenorrhea is abnormal and unhealthy for the body.

The following tips may help you resume menses or at least rule out nutrition-related factors.

1. **Throw away the bathroom scale**. Rather than striving to achieve a certain number on the scale, let your body weigh what it weighs. Focus on how healthy you feel and how well you perform rather than on the number you weigh.

2. **If you have weight to lose, don't crash-diet but rather moderately cut back on your food intake by about 20%.** Rapid weight loss may predispose you to amenorrhea. By following a healthy reducing program, such as outlined in chapter 17, you'll not only have greater success with long-term weight loss, but also have enough energy to run.

3. **If you are at an appropriate weight, practice eating as you did as a child.** Eat when you are hungry, stop when you are content. If you are always

hungry and are constantly obsessing about food, you are undoubtedly trying to eat too few calories. Chapter 13 can help you determine an appropriate calorie intake and eating schedule that may differ from your current routine, particularly if you yo-yo between starving and bingeing.

4. **Eat adequate protein.** Research has suggested that amenorrheic runners tend to eat less protein than their regularly menstruating counterparts. Even if you are a vegetarian, remember that you still need adequate protein (see chapter 7).

5. **Eat at least 20% of your calories from fat**. Runners commonly are afraid of eating fat, thinking if they eat fat, they'll get fat. Although excess calories from fat are easily fattening, some fat (20 to 30% of total calories) is an appropriate part of a healthy sports diet. (See chapter 8.)

6. **Maintain a calcium-rich diet to help maintain bone density.** Because you build peak bone density in your teens and early adult years, your goal is to protect against future problems with osteoporosis by including a serving of milk, yogurt, and other dairy or calcium-rich foods at each meal in the day. As I mentioned in chapter 1, a safe target is at least 1,000 mg of calcium per day if you are between 19 and 50 years old, and 1,200 mg of calcium per day if you are an amenorrheic or post-menopausal woman or a man over 50 years.

Steps to Resolve Eating Disorders

If you are spending too much time obsessing about food, weight and exercise, seek help and information on these websites:

- National Eating Disorders Association (information and referral network) www.NationalEatingDisorders.org
- American Dietetic Association (referral network) www.eatright.org
- Something Fishy Website on Eating Disorders (information and referral network) www.something-fishy.org
- Recommended self-help books www.EDcatalogue.com

If you suspect your training partner or friend is struggling with food issues, speak up! Anorexia and bulimia are self-destructive eating behaviors that may signal underlying depression and can be life threatening.

Here are some helpful tips:

- Approach the person gently but be persistent. Say that you are worried about her health. She, too, may be concerned about her loss of concentration, light-headedness, or chronic fatigue. These health changes are more likely to be a stepping-stone to accepting help, since the person clings to food and exercise for feelings of control and stability.
- Don't discuss weight or eating habits. Address the fundamental problems of life. Focus on unhappiness as the reason for seeking help. Point out what you see: ("I see you are very anxious. You look tired, are snappy, and easily irritated lately." Emphasize she doesn't have to be that way.
- Give her a list of resources (previously provided), and if you are really worried, make an appointment with a doctor, counselor, or sports dietitian and take her there yourself.

Remember that you are not responsible for resolving the eating issues and can only try to help. Your power comes from using community resources, eating disorders clinic, and health professionals.

"No matter what I do, I can't seem to stop gaining weight." Frustrated with her expanding waist, this former athlete, like others who are approaching menopause, is frightened about run-away weight gain. She started dieting and exercising harder to counter the flab and, over the din of the exercycle, asked, "Are women doomed to gain weight mid-life?" Here are the answers to some questions middle-aged women (and their husbands, children, and family members) commonly ask about weight and menopause.

Question: Do women inevitably gain fat with menopause?
No! Women do not always gain weight with menopause. Yes, women commonly get fatter and thicker around the middle as the fat settles in and around the abdominal area. But the changes are due more to lack of exercise and a surplus of calories than to a reduction of hormones. Young athletes with amennorhea (and reduced hormones) do not get fat.

In a three-year study with more than 3,000 women (initial age 42 to 52 years), the average weight gain was 4.6 pounds. The weight gain occurred in all women, regardless of their menopause status. (Sternfeld, Am J Epidemiol, 2004).

Question: If weight gain is not due to the hormonal shifts of menopause, what does cause it?

Here are a few culprits:
- Menopause occurs during a time of life when women may become less active. That is, if your children have grown up and left home, you may find yourself sitting more in front of a TV or computer screen, rather than running up and down stairs, carrying endless loads of laundry.
- A less active lifestyle not only reduces your calorie needs, but also results in a decline in muscle mass. Because muscle drives your metabolic rate, less muscle means a slower metabolism and fewer calories burned. (That is, of course, unless you wisely preserve your muscle by exercising.)
- Sleep patterns commonly change in mid-life. Add on top of that sleep-disrupting night sweats and a husband who snores, and many women end up feeling exhausted most of the time. Exhaustion and sleep deprivation can easily drain motivation to routinely exercise.
- Sleep deprivation is associated with weight gain. Adults who sleep less than seven hours per night tend to be heavier than their well-slept counterparts. When you are sleep deprived, your appetite grows. That is, the hormone that curbs your appetite (leptin) is reduced and the hormone that increases your appetite (grehlin) become more active. (Taheri, PLoS Med, 2004) Hence, you can have a hard time differentiating between "Am I tired?" or "Am I hungry?" You hear the cookie monster answer, "You're hungry and need many cookies...!"
- Menopause coincides with career success, including business meals at nice restaurants, extra wine, plush, vacations and cruises. Read that more calories and less exercise.
- By mid-life, most women are tired of dieting and depriving themselves of tempting foods; they may have been dieting since puberty! The "No, thank you" that prevailed at previous birthday parties now becomes "Yes, please."

Tips for Preventing Mid-Life Weight Gain and Optimizing Health

- The best way to prevent weight gain is to exercise and maintain an active lifestyle. Research suggests women who exercise do not the gain the weight and waist of their non-exercising peers (Sternfeld, Am J Epidem 2004). The exercise program should include both aerobic exercise (to enhance cardiovascular health) and strengthening exercise (to preserve muscle strength and bone density). The book *Strong Women Stay Thin* by Miriam Nelson is a good resource for developing a health-protective exercise program.
- Despite popular belief, taking hormones to counter the symptoms of menopause does not contribute to weight gain. If anything, hormone replacement therapy may help curb mid-life weight gain. (DiCarlo, Menopause, 2004).
- Menopausal women need a strong calcium intake: 1,200 mg calcium/day, or the equivalent of a serving of milk or yogurt at each meal. If you are tempted to take a supplement instead of consuming low-fat dairy foods, think again. One supplement does not replace the whole package of health-protective nutrients in low-fat milk and yogurt. Also, recent research suggests women who drink three or more servings of milk or yogurt per day tend to be leaner than milk-abstainers. Milk can help you lose—not gain—weight.
- If you have gained undesired fat, do not diet. If you have been dieting for 35 to 40 years of your adult life, you should have learned by now that dieting does not work. Rather, you need to learn how to eat healthfully. This means, fuel your body with enough breakfast, lunch and afternoon snack to curb your appetite (and energize your exercise program). Then, eat a lighter dinner. Think small calorie deficit. That is, consuming 100 fewer calories after dinner (theoretically) translates into losing 10 pounds of fat per year.
- To find peace with food and your body, meet with a registered dietitian (RD) who specializes in sports nutrition. This professional can develop a personalized food plan that fits your needs. To find a local RD, go to www.eatright.org or www.SCANdpg.org and enter your zip code into the referral network.

Also ask yourself: Am I really overweight? Maybe there is just more of you to love. Your body may not be quite as perfect as it once was at the height of your athletic career, but it can be good enough. I encourage you to focus on being fit and healthy, rather than being thin at any cost. No weight will ever do the enormous job of creating mid-life happiness.

For Skinny Runners: Preventing Undesired Weight Loss

If you are thin, and worried about becoming even leaner with added exercise, keep in mind that exercise tends to stimulate the appetite. Yes, a hard run may temporarily "kill" your appetite right after the workout because your body temperature is elevated. But within a few hours when you have cooled down, you will be plenty hungry. The more you exercise, the more you'll want to eat—assuming you make the time to do so. Here are a few tips to help you boost calories and prevent undesired weight loss.

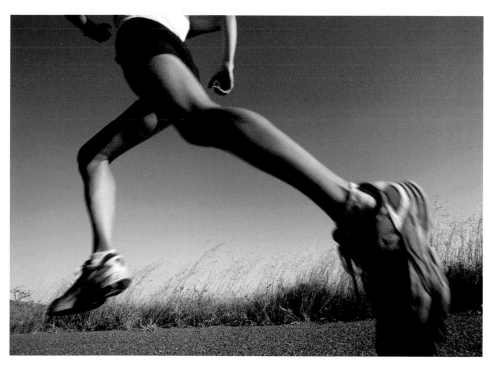

© Thinkstock/Stockbyte

Six Tips for Boosting Calories

1. Eat consistently.

Have at least three or four hearty meals plus one or two additional snacks daily.

Do not skip meals! You may not feel hungry for lunch if you've had a big breakfast, but you should eat regardless. Otherwise, you'll miss out on important calories that you need to accomplish your goal.

2. Eat larger portions.

Some runners think they need to buy expensive weight-gain powders. Not the case; standard foods work fine. The only reason commercial powders "work" is because they provide additional calories. For example, one runner religiously drank the recommended three glasses a day of a 300-calorie weight-gain shake; he consumed an extra 900 calories. Although he credited the protein shake for helping him manage his weight, he could have less expensively consumed those calories via supermarket foods.

I suggested that he simply eat larger portions of his standard fare:
- a bigger bowl of cereal
- a larger piece of fruit
- an extra sandwich for lunch
- two potatoes at dinner instead of one
- a taller glass of milk

When he did this, he met his goal of 1,000 extra calories per day and continued to see the desired results.

3. Select higher calorie foods, but not higher fat foods.

Excess fat calories easily convert into body fat that fattens you up rather than bulks up your muscles. The best bet for extra calories is to choose carbohydrate-dense foods that have more calories than an equally enjoyable counterpart (see chart in step 6). By reading food labels, you'll be able to make the best choices.

4. Drink lots of juice and low-fat milk.

Beverages are a simple way to increase your calorie intake. Replace part or all of the water you drink with calorie-containing fluids. (You don't need to drink water to get adequate water; juice is 99% water.) Extra juices are not only a great source of calories and fluids but also of carbohydrates to keep your muscles well fueled.

5. Do strength training (push-ups, weightlifting) to stimulate muscular development.

Strength training is essential if you want to bulk up (instead of fatten up). Resistance exercise is the key to muscular development.

6. Be patient.

If you are a scrawny high school or college student, your physique will undoubtedly fill out more easily as you get older. Know that you can be a strong runner by being well fueled and well trained. Your skinny legs may hurt your self-esteem more than your athletic ability.

Choose more:	Calories Amount	Instead of:	Calories Amount
Cranberry juice	170 8 oz (240 ml)	Orange juice	110 8 oz
Grape juice	160 8 oz (240 ml)	Grapefruit juice	100 8 oz
Banana	170 1 large	Apple	130 1 large
Granola	780 1.5 cups (150 g)	Bran flakes	200 1.5 cups (60 g)
Grape-Nuts	660 1.5 cups (175 g)	Cheerios	160 1.5 cups (45 g)
Corn	140 1 cup (165 g)	Green beans	40 1 cup (120 g)
Carrots	45 1 cup (150 g)	Zucchini	30 1 cup (180 g)
Split pea soup	130 1 cup (240 ml)	Vegetable soup	80 1 cup
Baked beans	260 1 cup (260 g)	Rice	190 1 cup (160 g)

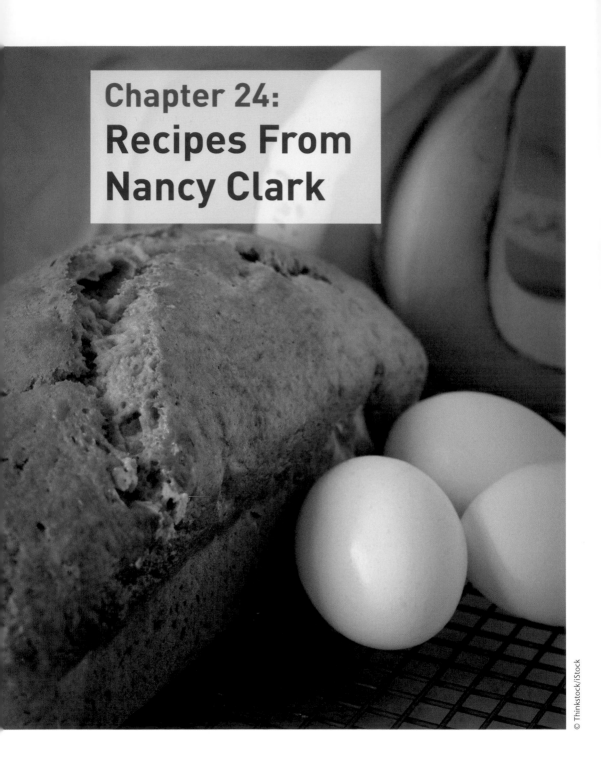

Chapter 24:
Recipes From Nancy Clark

© Thinkstock/iStock

Sweet Potato Fries

Sweet potato fries are yummy for dinner or even a snack. They offer a healthful way to satisfy your sweet tooth while fuelling your muscles with vitamin-rich carbs.

- 2 medium (1 pound; 0.5 kg) sweet potatoes or yams
- 2 tbsp (30 g) oil, preferably olive or canola
- 2 tbsp (25 g) brown sugar

1. Wash and thinly slice sweet potatoes into coin shapes.
2. Mix olive oil and brown sugar in a bowl. Add the sweet potatoes and mix well to coat the "coins."
3. Place them on a baking sheet lined with foil (for easy clean-up).
4. Bake at 425° F (220° C) for about 25 to 35 minutes, or until tender. Flip them half-way through baking.

Yield: 3 servings
Total calories: 750
Calories per serving: 250
42 g Carbohydrate
2 g Protein
8 g Fat

Recipe courtesy of Cat Whitehill. Reprinted with permission from *Food Guide for Soccer: Tips and Recipes From the Pros* by Gloria Averbuch and Nancy Clark.

Banana Bread

When you are confronted with bananas that are getting too ripe, consider making this recipe for banana bread. You'll enjoy it for a quick but hearty breakfast, lunch, or snack. Add some peanut butter and a glass of low-fat milk for a well-balanced meal and energy for the long run.

- 3 large bananas, the riper the better
- 1 egg or 2 egg whites
- 2 tbsp. (30 g) oil, preferably canola
- 1/3 to 1/2 cup (70-100 g) sugar
- 1/4 cup (60 ml) milk
- 1 tsp (5 g) salt, as desired
- 1 tsp (5 g) baking soda
- 1/2 tsp (2.3) baking powder
- 1 1/2 cups (180 g) flour, preferably half white, half whole-wheat

1. Preheat oven to 350°F (175°C).
2. Spray a 9x5-inch loaf pan with cooking spray.
3. In a large bowl, mash the bananas with a fork.
4. Add the egg, oil, sugar, milk, and salt. Beat well, and then add the baking soda and baking powder.
5. Gently blend the flour into the banana mixture. Stir for 20 seconds or until just moistened.
6. Pour the batter into the prepared pan.
7. Bake at 350°F (175°C) for 45 minutes or until a toothpick inserted near the middle comes out clean.

YIELD: 1 loaf, 12 slices **Total calories:** 1,600 **Calories per slice:** 140
Carbodydrate 24 g, Protein 3 g, Fat 3 g

From: *Nancy Clark's Sport Nutrition Guidebook*, Fourth Edition (Human Kinetics, 2008)

A Super Salad

A colorful salad is a super way to boost your nutrient intake! Here's a suggestion for a super salad that is rich in not only vitamins, but also in protein (to build muscles), carbs (to fuel muscles), fiber (to move food through your system), and healthful fats and phytochemicals to help fight inflammation.

By eating a portfolio of nutrient-dense foods at most meals, you need not rely on vitamin pills to compensate for lousy eating.

In a large bowl, combine your choice of colorful salad vegetables, such as:
- Spinach
- Tomato
- Red pepper
- Yellow pepper
- Carrot

Add protein and healthful fat:
- Flaked Tuna
- Tofu cubes
- Chickpeas
- Kidney beans
- Cottage cheese, low-fat
- Shredded cheese, low-fat
- Walnuts or almonds, chopped
- Avocado slices
- Olive oil-based salad dressing

Accompany with your choice of wholesome carbs:
- Whole-wheat English muffin
- Toasted whole-grain bread
- Fresh rolls
- Whole-grain crackers

Turkey Burgers

Ground turkey is a leaner alternative to ground beef. But leaner can sometimes mean "dry and tasteless."

This recipe yields a tasty, juicy turkey burger that you'll want to enjoy time and again.

- 1/2 cup (30 g) uncooked oatmeal
- 1/2 cup (240 ml) turkey or chicken broth (canned), or milk
- 1 pound (450 g) ground turkey
- 1 egg or two egg whites
- 1 small onion, grated or finely chopped
- **Optional:** salt, pepper, two dashes of nutmeg

1. In a medium bowl, combine the oatmeal, broth or milk, egg or egg whites, onion, and seasonings.
2. Add the ground turkey, mix well, and then shape into 4 patties.
3. Cook over medium heat in a nonstick skillet for about 5 minutes per side.

Yield: 4 patties
Total calories: 750
Calories per serving: 190
Carbohydrate: 5 g
Protein: 26 g
Fat: 7 g

Cheesecake Snackwiches

While standard cheesecake is a nutritional nightmare, this healthier alternative offers the same flavor but with less saturated fat.

These snackwiches are easy to make, and a nice treat for a dessert or afternoon energizer. Graham crackers are considered a whole grain, so this is one tasty way to boost your whole grain intake.

- 2 graham cracker squares
- 1 tsp (5 g) low-fat cream cheese
- 1 tsp (5 g) jam
- **Optional:** sprinkling of cinnamon

1. Spread 1 graham cracker with low-fat cream cheese.
2. Add the jam; sprinkle with cinnamon, if desired.
3. Top with the second graham cracker, making into a sandwich. Enjoy!

Total calories: 90 (if you can eat just one!)
Carbohydrate: 16 g
Protein: 2 g
Fat 2 g

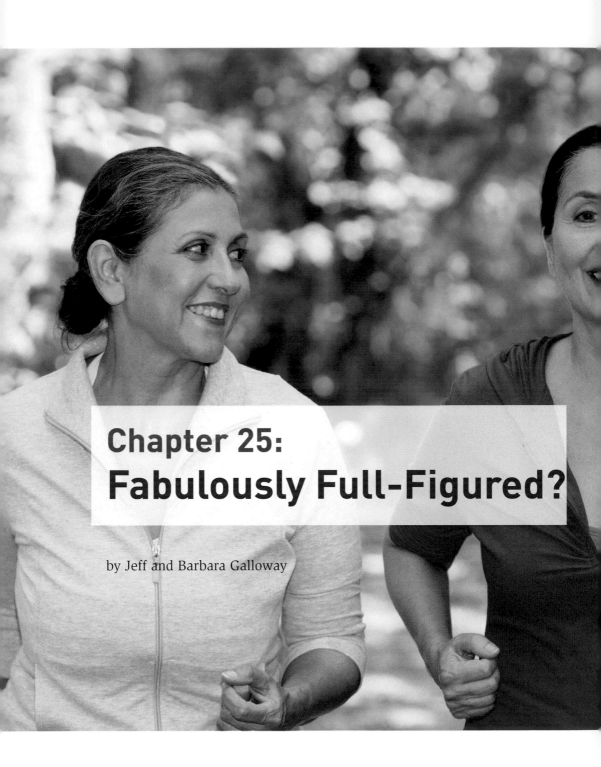

Chapter 25:
Fabulously Full-Figured?

by Jeff and Barbara Galloway

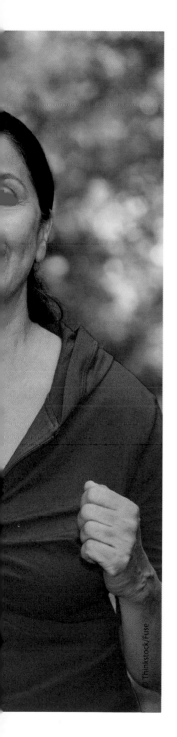

Thinkstock/Fuse

While we were writing this book, a growing number of women who are larger than the average person, asked for a chapter dealing with some special issues. After consulting with a variety of those who have fought these battles and are still doing so successfully, the following information is offered—with inspirational stories. Some of the stories involve women who started using walking as exercise, but got into running. You can choose the type of exercise you wish—don't give up!

85 Pounds Light and Counting

Tracy B added the usual weight during her pregnancy, and kept on going. When the scales told her that she was almost 100 pounds over her healthy weight, she walked out the door and kept going. A local charity marathon team provided her with a cause and good friends, as she walked her way to the marathon. "The marathon team I became a part of is like a little extension of my family." Instead of trying a restrictive diet, she simply tried reasonable sized meals and no high-fat snacks. She's still 10 pounds from her goal, but is still losing.

"Don't look at the big number of pounds you need to lose. Set an attainable goal, maybe 10 pounds at a time. And if you fall off the wagon, get back on and don't beat yourself up about it. Be proud of how hard you are working."

Tips From Tracy

1. Never give up on yourself and be very proud of yourself for any effort you're making to make yourself healthier and fit.
2. Don't beat yourself up for "falling off the wagon"—this will happen at some point. Just dust yourself off and make that day your first day again—don't look back!
3. Don't let friends or family members discourage your efforts. I know this sounds odd because these people should be your support system, but some people don't adapt to change very well and can feel threatened by the new you and your new group of friends.
4. Eat a very healthy, well-balanced diet. If you're not sure how to get started with this either consult this book or check with your doctor or nutritionist.
5. Then make yourself a fat-burning machine. When I first started walking I would walk on my breaks at work, my lunch hour, and then do my regular distance when I got home.
6. Be sure to cross-train. Not only is this good for your muscles, but it's good for your brain, too.
   You deserve your time to exercise!
7. I think the biggest thing for women (no matter what size) is that **you deserve to give this to yourself.** My job and my family get me for 14 out of the 16 hours I put in a day. I allow myself to take those other two hours for me—guilt free! I need this—distance walking defines who I am. In return, my family gets a healthier and happier Mom! I want to be around to see my kids grow up and then run circles around my grandkids!

Tips From Sherry: More Than 150 Pounds Lost...Runs Marathons

Exercise was the theme in rising out of depression and into a vigorous life. Be sure to read her moving and inspirational story in chapter 98. Here are her points:

- If you are considerably overweight, see your doctor, and get shoes from a good running store.
- Winded when doing even gentle exercise? Then walk slowly at first.
- Excess skin—Use girdles, spandex, knee-to-chest Flexee that keeps it from getting in the way.
- Back issues: Physical therapy can help. Ab strengthening helped a bit. The only thing that ultimately helped me was getting my excess skin removed after weight loss. Don't lean over or look down—stay upright!
- Make sure to shower and dry off properly. Excess skin and moisture is a prime habitat for a yeast infection.
- Larger women feel self-conscious when exercising. Ladies-only full-service gyms are a good supportive environment to get started. I found that my fellow runners are really nice people no matter how much faster they are than you. As heavy as I was, I always got friendly waves and greetings on the running trails. Be proud, don't look down!
- Don't be afraid of your first race. Most races have a big walking group. Sign up with friends".

Bras

Be prepared to pay significantly more than you would pay for your everyday bra—sometimes as much as you would pay for your shoes. Remember that bras usually last a lot longer than shoes.

There are a growing number of bras designed for specific types of exercise, based upon cup size. Many large-breasted women have reported success with the Enell brand and the Fiona model from Moving Comfort. Champion has a seamless underbra with underwire that has also been successful.

- Many of the well-constructed "workout bras" are not supportive for runners. The elastic in these products (for twisting and extraneous motion in tennis, Pilates) allows for significant bouncing and stress when running.
- Comfort: Look first at the fibers next to your skin. The microfibers can move moisture away from your skin, reducing chaffing (see next section), moisture chill, and weight increase due to the absorption of sweat by cotton and similar fibers.
- C, D, and E cups: More support is needed. Look for a bra that will fit each breast, and a strap that has minimal or no elastic. The best placement of the straps will differ among individuals—so try on a variety of bras to find the configuration that matches up with your body. If you receive pressure on the shoulders, where the straps press down, padded straps can help.

Exercise improves health and well-being—even when obese. This is the finding of numerous studies at the Cooper Research Institute (Dallas, Texas) and other institutions. At Cooper, the obese-but-fit subjects were shown to have a healthier profile than sedentary thin subjects.

Worried about the way they look in public, many heavier women don't exercise. That's too bad because it is clear that even 10 minutes of regular movement of the feet will bestow a better attitude, and can lead to higher self-esteem. Short exercise segments will also burn fat! It is easier to piece together several segments of 100-200 steps than 30 minutes at one time. Smaller segments tend to reduce appetite increase in most of the exercisers that we've heard from on the issue.

Read chapter 13—The set point mechanism can help you understand fat deposition, and what you can do to hold your own—or lower it. And please, don't go on a restrictive diet. These usually produce water loss and increased fat accumulation and more weight, after the diet has ended.

Low-carb diets don't tell you this....

- The weight loss is usually water loss, with glycogen loss.
- Almost everyone on this diet resumes regular eating, within a few weeks or months.
- Almost all low-carb dieters gain back more weight than they lost.
- You lose the energy and motivation to exercise.
- You lose exercise capacity that can help to keep the weight off when you resume eating normally.
- Your metabolism rate goes down—making it harder to keep the weight off.

Group support is huge—Join or start a charity fund-raising or training group, such as that for www.BreastCancerMarathon.com. The programs at Weight Watchers and Curves can be very successful because of group support. For Galloway Training Groups, visit www.JeffGalloway.com.

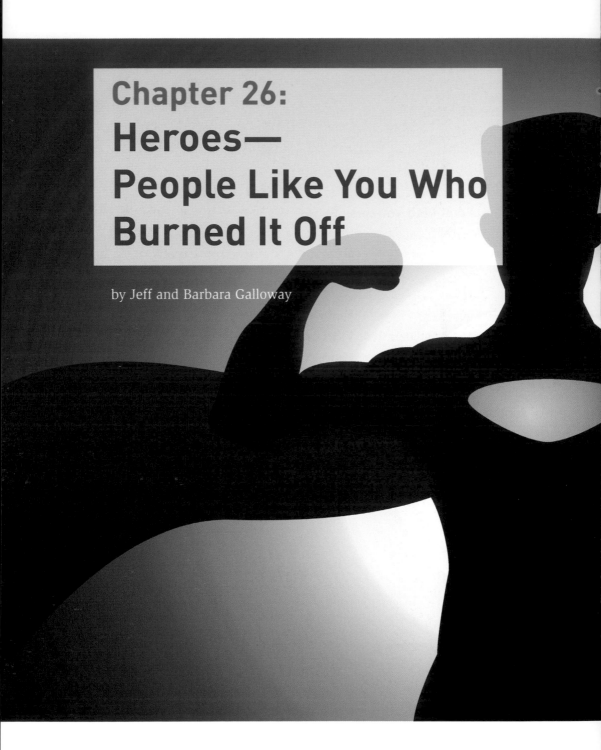

Chapter 26:
Heroes—
People Like You Who
Burned It Off

by Jeff and Barbara Galloway

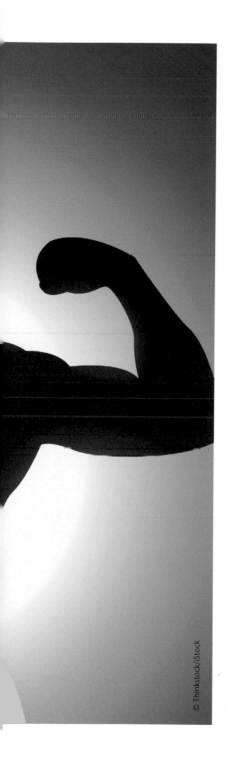

© Thinkstock/iStock

98 Pounds Off...And Still Losing

Karen had been overweight most of her life, and, as she puts it "definitely not athletic." But she had taken the path used by women through the ages: "I had tried every diet, spent an embarrassing amount of money on diet programs." The weight would drop for a few weeks or months and then, steadily rise until it surpassed the pre-diet amount. For some reason, surpassing 200, 225 and 250, pounds was OK. When the nurse told her she weighed 271, she held it in until reaching her car and then the tears flowed.

When her friend Jo decided to train for the Country Music Half Marathon (Nashville), Karen was determined to use this race as a goal to be an every-other-day walker. Her fitness improved week by week; she found the challenge of this 13-miler highly motivating. The run-walk-run method allowed her to move from a walker to a runner. So, in her late 30s, weighing 230 pounds, Karen ran a minute and walked a minute. Sedentary spouse Paul was so impressed by her steady progress that he began running also, at 278 pounds. Two years later, Paul had lost 90 pounds. Karen has lost 98 pounds and is still losing. As Karen approached the finish line of the Country Music 13.1-miler, the tears started flowing again—for all of the right reasons. Karen and Paul schedule vacations around running events now, and get stressed when they cannot run.

"If you're a beginner, start with short run-walk intervals. It's better to set realistic goals that you can meet and then adjust them as you improve."

145 Pounds Lighter

"I have traded my addiction to food for an addiction to running. I truly believe running has allowed me to cope with the mental and physical stresses of daily life, motherhood, and work more effectively."
Angela was an overweight kid from an obese family. By the age of 35, she weighed 280 pounds with high blood pressure, and back, knee, and hip pain. She also had a serious gastric reflux problem, and surgery was recommended.

In January of 2005, after months of psychological counseling and exercise (primarily walking and elliptical), she had the gastric bypass operation. She soon discovered that surgery doesn't change a genetic predisposition to obesity, nor the desire to cope with stress by overeating (many patients gain back some of their weight after these surgeries). Because of her surgery, she had to eat less and avoid certain foods because of their physical side effects.

Having enjoyed the stress relief of the pre-operation exercise, Angela continued to walk. Six months later, and 85 pounds lighter, she decided to "step it up" by inserting some short running segments into her walks and completed a 10K and then a half marathon during the training season. By this time she had lost a total of 120 pounds, crediting running with "revving up" the fat burning.

Looking for some guidance, she joined our Galloway Training program, finished the Richmond Marathon, and set her sights on the "original" marathon in Athens, Greece. Despite some health setbacks during the training, she kept improving endurance and lost another 25 pounds. On the difficult Greek course (with a 13-mile hill), Angela set a new personal record by 22 minutes!

Kathryn Lost Over 100 Pounds: Portion Control and Marathon Training

"To lose it and keep it off it has to be a lifestyle change, whether it is 30 pounds or 100 pounds. It also has to come from your heart that you want to do it."

Even when Kathryn was severely obese and had trouble jogging a few steps, she had a vision that she could become a marathoner. At first, it took her 25 minutes to cover a mile. At this pace, she would not be allowed to continue in the race, because the course would have been closed—and she had 25 more miles to go! While many would have given up, Kathryn got moving. At first, she set her sights on one mile at a time and one pound at a time—then, one week at a time.

In spite of the fatigue she experienced during marathon training, Kathryn discovered an infusion of motivation from inside.

Here are some of her tips:
* A short term goal seems easier to reach.
* Once you reach that goal immediately set another one.
* Advising others to train for a goal was so motivating—help others while helping yourself.
* When you are coming toward the finish line, look at it as a start—improving the rest of your life.

- I didn't want to cut out foods that I liked. So I ate them, but I cut the portion.
- Food in gives fuel for walking and running.
- Walking and running burned off the fat—a little bit each week.

"What kept me going? I knew how good I was feeling inside, what I was doing for my health. I felt stronger. If your goal is to finish a marathon, then do it, but don't stop!"

Sherry Began Her Journey at 348 Pounds—And Has Lost More Than 150 Pounds (See her tips in chapter 25.)

"A normal 25-year-old female should be happy, healthy, and full of life. At 25 I was lazy, super obese, unhealthy, depressed, and had minimal self-confidence. I always had a weight problem: 40 pounds overweight at 15, 70 pounds at 18. By the time I graduated college and married at age 22, I was an incredible 125 pounds overweight, and at my 25th birthday, I weighed 348 pounds!

"I cannot pinpoint one reason that led me to being super obese with a BMI of 56. I did not have an easy time growing up. My older sister was gravely ill when I was young, and my mom had a difficult time dealing with depression and anxiety. At times I felt like I was not loved, which led to sexual abuse as a teenager. I was diagnosed with Polycystic Ovarian Syndrome (PCOS), which results in fertility problems and heightened levels of insulin resistance. I loved to eat carbs, which really packed on the pounds. It was an atrocious cycle— the more I would eat, the less I could exercise. The heavier I got, the more I became depressed, which led me to eating more to comfort myself."

My Breaking Point—"My husband and I tried to start a family for months, with no success. Hormone therapy didn't work either and triggered hair loss in clumps, mood swings, and hot flashes. I was miserable. Finally, we were scheduled to see a reproductive endocrinologist but were then rejected because I was too heavy and the pregnancy risks to me and the baby would be too great. I knew that I was on track for a heart attack, and I loved my husband too much to leave him tragically at a young age."

"My Decision to change my life started with a gastric bypass operation. I lost weight quickly and easily because my stomach was now the size of an egg. My new stomach was a tool, and being successful at weight loss would be a life-long commitment. As soon as I was released from the hospital I began an exercise regimen, mall walking and a ladies-only gym. The exercise was helping to keep the fat off. Then, my friend Susan won an entry in the Peachtree Road Race, the world's largest 10K. I thought anyone who could run a 5K was an elite athlete! I was in awe when she finished the race in 80 minutes. Then came the great visualization: If she could do it, then so can I!"

Ready, Set, Go! "There was no starting gun to signal the start of my training, but I sure was fired up. I set a goal of running in the Kaiser Permanente Corporate 5K, just over a month away. The night before the race I woke up in horrible pain at 2 a.m. My husband rushed me to the ER where they discovered I had a hole somewhere in my digestive system. I had emergency surgery, which led to a 14-inch scar, 40 staples, and a week's vacation at Gwinnett Medical Center. I was distraught. I felt that everything I worked hard to achieve was ruined. I cried for three hours straight. The nurses tried to make me feel better, but I was inconsolable. At this point, my only dream was shattered.
A week after being released from the hospital, I started walking, even with pain. I signed up for a local 10K, trained, and finished—I was a runner! I immediately found my husband and announced I wanted to run a marathon. He pretty much thought I was insane, but I joined a training group, dealt with the gastric/fluid absorption problems, excessive loose skin, and back pain. I crossed the Chicago Marathon finish line and a wave of emotions overcame me. At 348 pounds, I never once imagined being able to run to my mailbox. Through many trials and tribulation, and mostly hard work, I was able to lose the weight and do what I once thought was unthinkable."

Through sweat, hard work, and even a few tears I was able to accomplish each of the goals I set for myself because I developed a strong mental attitude and took charge over my health and fitness. I had the seeds of these capabilities when I was a depressed 348-pounder—and didn't know it. You do, too."

Overcoming an Eating Disorder

Julie was an overweight child, rode horses, ate pop tarts and tater tots, had a wonderful Mom, but experienced self-esteem issues. As a 9th grader (180 pounds, 5' 10") she broke her foot falling off a horse, hobbled around and got depressed, and reduced her quantity of food. As she lost weight, she received positive feedback from peers for the first time in her life ("You look good"), and started to feel good about herself. So she ate even less and lost more—down to 110 lbs!

"I don't remember when, or how, but I noticed things starting to change. I was still getting attention, but it was from those with concern. I started riding again and my trainer approached me and asked me to feel free to come to her if I had a problem because she had been there before. I started feeling light-headed all the time, I would try to stand up and literally fall right back down. I quit getting my period, and it was a struggle to walk, let alone ride. Bottom line was that I felt weak, and I knew I needed to do something about it."

She started running and walking (alternating mailboxes) but was so hungry and weak that she ate more, became energetic and felt strong, settling into a healthy weight of 145 pounds. Then came college. Caring for horses, studying hard, commuting to school took time, and she stopped running. "My mind went into a hard downward spiral of self-esteem once again, and I started something new, turning to food for comfort. I didn't do drugs or smoke, but I turned to food for that quick endorphin boost. I would find myself tired, frustrated, and disgusted, and would lock myself in my room literally gorging on whatever was in sight." The scales exceeded the 200 mark, she hated herself, and hid from friends.

"I wrote in a diary every night about how I would change, only to fail the following day. Again, I had hit a very low point and knew I needed to do something. Knowing I could not control my eating habits, I started trying to control something I knew I could, my exercise. I started running again. And again, experienced the same psychological response as I did in high school. I felt better about myself, I started to lose weight, and I was able to pull myself out of the slump."

Julie was inspired: to read about proper nutrition, to eat more meals each day, and to train for a marathon. "My mood sailed and I could conquer the world, or could I? I trained (running straight out) to the point of completing my first half marathon, which sent me to straight burn out. My runs became a constant struggle, and I started to hate every second of them. I stopped running, and up went the weight, down went the self-esteem and mood."

Julie fell in love, with Chris, and they decided to train for a marathon. "I stumbled across the most wonderful concept, something that up until now my body had known but I did not, *eating gave you fuel.*"

She started running stronger and faster and broke all of her personal records.

"I no longer run because I eat too much; I eat so that I can run. I have dropped weight, but my body composition has completely changed. My body fat is the lowest it has ever been, and guess what, I'm eating Reese's Peanut Butter Cups and white breads! Who would have thought?"

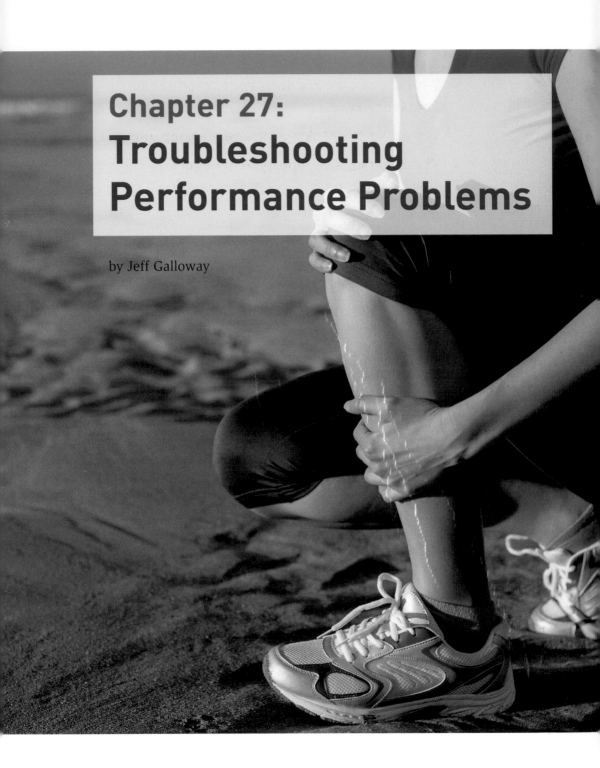

Chapter 27:
Troubleshooting Performance Problems

by Jeff Galloway

Pace and motivation slows at end of races:

- **You did not eat enough of your blood sugar booster snacks.**

- **You didn't start taking the snacks soon enough.**

- **You didn't eat the right type of sugar.**

- **You didn't drink a small amount of water with the snacks.**

- **Your long runs aren't long enough.**

- **You are running too fast at the beginning of the race.**

- **You may benefit from walk breaks that are taken more frequently.**

- **You may be overtrained—back off the speed sessions for a week or two.**

- **In track workouts, run hardest at the end of the workout.**

- **Temperature or humidity may be to blame—try slowing down at the beginning.**

Pace and motivation slows in the middle of the race:

- You didn't start your blood sugar boosting snack early enough.
- You didn't eat enough calories or eat frequently enough.
- You may be running too hard at the beginning—slow down by a few seconds each mile.
- You may benefit from more frequent walk breaks.

Nauseous at the end:

- You ate too much of your blood sugar snack during the race.
- You ate food that was too hard to digest.
- You drank too much during the run.
- You consumed an electrolyte beverage during the run.
- You ran too fast at the beginning or the middle.
- Temperature is above 65°F/17°C.
- You ate too much (or drank too much) before the race or workout—even hours before.
- You ate the wrong foods—most commonly, fat, fried foods, milk products, fibrous foods.
- Low blood sugar can result in nausea.

Tired during workouts:

- You didn't keep your blood sugar level boosted before the run.
- You didn't eat regular blood sugar boosting snacks during the run.
- The snacks during did not have enough simple carbohydrate.
- You did a poor job of refueling after finishing your last run.
- You are low in B vitamins.
- You are low in iron—have a serum ferritin test.
- You are not eating enough protein.
- You are eating too much fat—especially before or right after a run.
- You are running too many days per week.
- You are running too hard on long runs.
- Running too hard on all running days.
- You are not taking enough walk breaks from the beginning of your runs.
- You allow insufficient rest days between hard workouts.

Side Pain

This is very common and usually has a simple fix. Normally it is nothing to worry about…it just hurts. This condition is due to 1) the lack of lower lung breathing, and 2) going a little too fast from the beginning of the run. You can correct #2 easily by slowing your pace during the first mile or two.

Lower lung breathing from the beginning of a run can prevent side pain. This way of inhaling air is performed by diverting the air you breathe into your lower lungs. Also called *belly breathing*, this is how we breathe when asleep, and it provides maximum opportunity for oxygen absorption. If you don't breathe this way when you run, and you are not getting the oxygen you need, the side pain will tell you. By slowing down, walking, and breathing deeply for a while, the pain may go away. But sometimes it does not. Most runners just continue to run and walk with the side pain. In 50 years of running and helping others run, I've not seen any lasting negative effect from those who run with a side pain—it just hurts.

You don't have to take in a maximum breath to perform this technique. Simply breathe a normal breath but send it to the lower lungs. You know that you have done this if your stomach goes up and down as you inhale and exhale. If your chest goes up and down, you are breathing shallowly.

Note: Consuming too much food or fluid before a run will inhibit lower lung breathing and can cause a side pain.

I Feel Great One Day...And Not the Next

If you can solve this problem, you could become a very wealthy person. There are a few common reasons for this, but there will always be "those days" when the body doesn't seem to work right, or the gravity seems heavier than normal—and you cannot find a reason. You should keep looking for the causes of this, using your journal. If you feel this way several times a week, for two or more weeks in a row, you may need more rest in your program.

1. Low blood sugar can make any run a bad run. You may feel good at the start and suddenly feel like you have no energy. Every step seems to take a major effort.
2. Just do it. In most cases, this is a one-day occurrence. Most runners just put more walking into the mix, slow down, and get through it. Before doing a speed workout, however, make sure that there's not a medical reason for the "bad" feeling. I've had some of my best workouts after feeling very bad during the first few miles—or the first few speed repetitions.
3. Heat or humidity will make you feel worse. You will often feel better when the temperature is below 60°F and miserable when 75°F or above—or the humidity is high. If it is above 70°F on a mile repeat day, do twice as many 800s instead, walking 3 minutes between each.
4. Low motivation. Use the rehearsal techniques in chapter 1 to get you out the door on a bad day. These have helped numerous runners turn their minds around—even in the middle of a run.
5. Infection can leave you feeling lethargic, achy, and unable to run at the same pace that was easy a few days earlier. Check the normal signs (fever, chills, swollen lymph glands, higher morning pulse rate) and at least call your doctor if you suspect something.
6. Medication and alcohol, even when taken the day before, can leave a hangover that doesn't affect any area of your life except for your running. Your doctor or pharmacist should be able to tell you about the effect of medication on strenuous exercise.
7. A slower start can make the difference between a good day and a bad day. When your body is on the edge of fatigue or other stress, it only takes a

few seconds too fast per mile, walking or running, to push into discomfort or worse. A quick adjustment to a slightly slower pace before you get too tired can turn this around.

8. Caffeine can help because it gets the central nervous system working to top capacity. I feel better and my legs work so much better when I have had a cup of coffee an hour before the start of a run. Of course, those who have problems with caffeine should avoid it—or consult a doctor.

Cramps in the Muscles

At some point, most people who run will experience an isolated cramp. These muscle contractions usually occur in the feet or the calf muscles and may come during a run or walk, or they may hit at random afterward. Most commonly, they will occur at night, or when you are sitting around at your desk or watching TV in the afternoon or evening. When severe cramps occur during a run, you will have to stop or significantly slow down.

Cramps vary in severity. Most are mild but some can grab so hard that they shut down the muscles and hurt when they seize up. Massage, and a short and gentle movement of the muscle can help to bring most of the cramps around. Odds are that stretching will make the cramp worse, or tear the muscle fibers.

Sometimes a buffered salt tablet can reduce the chance of cramps. However, most cramps are due to overuse—doing more than in the recent past, or continuing to put yourself at your limit, especially in warm weather. Look at the pace and distance of your runs and workouts in your training journal to see if you have been running too far, too fast, or both. If the muscle is exhausted and you continue to push the effort, no salt tablet can help.

• Continuous running increases cramping. Taking walk breaks more often can reduce or eliminate them. Several runners who used to cramp when they ran continuously, stopped cramping with a 10- to 30-second walk every three to five minutes during a long or fast run.

• During hot weather, enjoy some salty foods (pretzels, broth, salt sprinkled on oatmeal) before your exercise to help retain water in your body. Dehydration can be associated with muscle cramping.

- On very long runs, however, the continuous sweating, especially when drinking a lot of fluid (more than 20 oz an hour), can push your sodium levels too low and produce muscle cramping. If this happens regularly, a buffered salt tablet has helped greatly—a product like Succeed! If you have any blood pressure or other sodium issues, check with your doctor first.
- Many medications, especially those designed to lower cholesterol, have as one of their known side effects, muscle cramps. Runners who use medications and cramp should ask their doctor if there are alternatives.

Here are several ways of dealing with cramps:

- Take a longer and more gentle warm-up.
- Shorten your run segment—or take walk breaks more often.
- Slow down your walk, and walk more.
- Break your run up into two segments (not on long runs or speed workouts).
- Look at any other exercise that could be causing the cramps.
- Eat salty foods or take a buffered salt tablet at the beginning of your exercise.
- Form issues: Don't push off as hard, or bounce as high off the ground.
- During speed workouts on hot days, walk more during the rest interval.
- Ensure adequate fluid consumption during exercise.

Note: If you have high blood pressure or similar problem, ask your doctor before taking any salt product.

Upset Stomach or Diarrhea

Sooner or later, virtually every runner has at least one episode with nausea or diarrhea. It comes from the build-up of total stress that you accumulate in your life—and specifically the stress of the workout. But stress is the result of many unique conditions within the individual. Your body produces the nausea or diarrhea to get you to reduce the exercise, which will reduce the stress. Here are the common causes.

1. Running too fast or too far Is the most common cause. Runners are confused about this, because the pace doesn't feel too fast in the beginning. Each person has a level of fatigue that triggers these conditions. Slowing down and taking more walk breaks will help you manage the problem. Speed training and racing will increase stress very quickly.

2. Eating too much or too soon before the run. Your system has to work hard when running, and it is also hard work to digest food. Doing both at the same time raises stress and results in nausea. Having food in your stomach, in the process of being digested is an extra stress and a likely target for elimination.

3. Eating a high-fat or high-protein diet. Even one meal that has over 50% of the calories in fat or protein can lead to nausea or diarrhea hours later.

4. Eating too much the afternoon or evening the day before. A big evening meal will still be in the gut the next morning, being digested. When you bounce up and down on a run, which you will, you add stress to the system, sometimes resulting in nausea or diarrhea.

5. Heat and humidity are a major cause of these problems. Some people don't adapt well to even modest heat increases and experience nausea or diarrhea when racing (or doing speed sessions) at the same pace that did not produce the problem in cool weather. In hot conditions, everyone has a core body temperature increase that will result in significant stress to the system—often causing nausea, and sometimes diarrhea. By slowing down, taking more walk breaks, and pouring water over your head, you can manage this better.

6. Drinking too much water before a run. If you have too much water in your stomach, and you are bouncing around, you put stress on the digestive system. Reduce your intake to the bare minimum. Most runners don't need to drink any fluid before a run that is 60 minutes or less.

7. Drinking too much of a sugar or electrolyte drink. Water is the easiest substance for the body to process. The addition of sugar or electrolyte minerals, as in a sports drink, makes the substance harder to digest. During a run (especially on a hot day) it is best to drink only water if you have had nausea, diarrhea, or other problems. Cold water is best.

Note: Drinking too little fluid during a long run can lead to diarrhea.

8. Drinking too much fluid (especially a sugar drink) too soon after a run. Even if you are very thirsty, don't gulp down large quantities of any fluid during a short period of time. Try to drink no more than 6-8 oz, every 20 minutes or so. If you are particularly prone to nausea, diarrhea, just take two to four sips, every five minutes or so. When the body is very stressed and tired, it's not a good idea to consume a sugar drink (sports drink). The extra stress of digesting the sugar can lead to problems.

9. Don't let running be stressful to you. Some runners get too obsessed about getting their run in or running at a specific pace. This adds stress to your life. Relax and let your run diffuse some of the other tensions in your life. When you are under a lot of life stress it's OK to delay a speed workout when the thought of fast running seems to increase your stress level. Take an easy jog!

10. Pay attention to daily bowel issues. Problems during the day can be increased during a run.

Headache

There are several reasons why runners get headaches on runs. While uncommon, they happen to the average runner about one to five times a year. The extra stress that running puts on the body can trigger a headache on a tough day—even considering the relaxation that comes from the run. Many runners find that a dose of an over-the-counter headache medication takes care of the problem. As always, consult with your doctor about use of medication. Here are the causes and their solutions.

Dehydration—If you run in the morning, make sure that you hydrate well the day before. Avoid alcohol the night before if you run in the mornings and have headaches.

Medications can often produce dehydration—There are some medications that make runners more prone to headaches. Check with your doctor.

Too hot for you—Run at a cooler time of the day (usually in the morning before the sun gets above the horizon). When on a hot run, pour water over your head.

Being in the sun—Try to stay in the shade as much as possible. Wear a visor not a hat, making sure the band is not too tight.

Running a little too fast—Start all runs more slowly, walk more during the first half of the run.

Low blood sugar level—Be sure that you boost your BLS with a snack, about 30 minutes before you run. If you are used to having it, caffeine in a beverage can sometimes help this situation also—but caffeine causes headaches for a small percentage of runners.

If prone to migranes—Generally avoid caffeine, and try your best to avoid dehydration. Talk to your doctor about other possibilities.

Watch your neck and lower back—If you have a slight forward lean as you run, you can put pressure on the spine—particularly in the neck and lower back. Read the form chapter in this book and see if running upright doesn't help the problem.

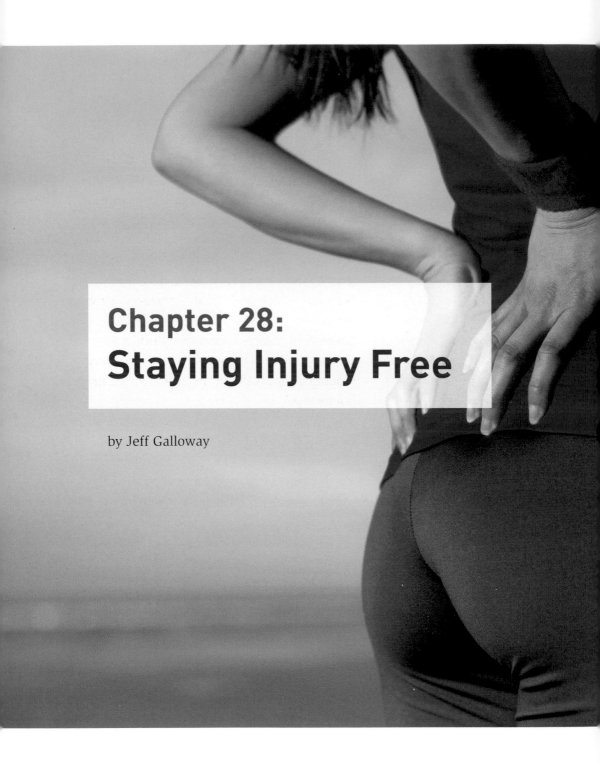

Chapter 28:
Staying Injury Free

by Jeff Galloway

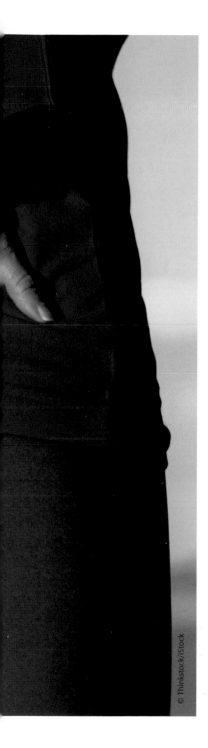

© Thinkstock/iStock

Note: For more information in this area, see the book *Running Injuries* by Jeff Galloway and Dr. David Hannaford. It is available at www.JeffGalloway.com.

Because running and walking are activities that enabled our ancient ancestors to survive, we have the ability to adapt to these two patterns of motion if we use these principles:

- Walk or run at a gentle pace—and insert walk breaks from the beginning.
- Schedule sufficient rest between each workout.
- Exercise regularly—about every other day.
- When increasing exercise, do so very gradually, and reduce the intensity of the longer workout.
- The single greatest reason for improvement in running is *not getting injured.*

But inside each human is a personality trait that can compromise exercise enjoyment. I call this the "Type A overworker syndrome." Those who are candidates for Boston are prime candidates. When the workload is a bit too much, the body responds to the challenge at first. When the runner keeps pushing, without enough rest between, the body breaks at one of the weak links. Here are some guidelines given as one exerciser to another.

Be sensitive to weak links.

Each of us has a very few areas that take on more stress, and tend to register most of the aches, pains, and injuries. The most common sites are the knees, the feet, the shins, and the hips. If you have a particular place on your knee that has been hurt before, and it hurts during or after exercise, take extra days off, and follow the suggestions concerning treating an injury, listed next.

How do you know that you are injured?

The following are the leading signs that you have an injury. If you feel any of the three, you should stop your workout immediately and take some extra rest days (at least 2 days). Continuing to do the same exercise that irritated the tendon or muscle at the early stages of an injury creates a dramatically worse injury—even during one workout. If you take two to three days off at the first symptom, you may avoid having to stop exercise for two to three months by trying to push through the pain. It is always safer to err on the side of taking more time off when you first notice one of the following:

1. **Inflammation**—any type of swelling
2. **Loss of function**—the knee, foot, or other area doesn't work correctly
3. **Pain**—that does not go away when you walk for a few minutes

Losing conditioning.

Studies have shown that you can maintain conditioning even when you don't run for five days. Surely you want to continue regular exercise if you can, but staying injury free has an even higher priority. So don't be afraid to take up to five days off when a "weak link" kicks in. In most cases you will only stop for two to three days.

Treatment

It is always best at the first sign of a real injury to see a doctor (or with muscle injury—a massage therapist) who wants to get you exercising again as soon as possible. The better doctors will explain what they believe is wrong (or tell you when they cannot come up with a diagnosis) and give you a treatment plan. This will give you great confidence in the process, which has been shown to speed the healing.

Treatments while you are waiting to see a doctor.

Unfortunately, most of the better doctors are so booked up that it may take several days and sometimes weeks to see them. While waiting for your appointment, here are some things other exercisers have done when one of the weak links kicks in:

- Take two to five days off from any activity that could irritate it.
- If the area is next to the skin (tendon, foot, etc), rub a chunk of ice on the area—constantly rubbing for 15 minutes until the area gets numb. Continue to do this for a week after you feel no symptoms. The chunk of ice must be rubbed constantly and directly on the tissue where the injury is located. (Ice bags and gel ice do virtually nothing).
- If the problem is inside a joint or muscle, call your doctor and ask if you can use prescription strength anti-inflammatory medication. Don't take any medication without a doctor's advice—and follow that advice.
- If you have a muscle injury, see a very successful sports massage therapist. Find one who has a lot of successful experience treating the area where you are injured. The magic fingers and hands can often work wonders.
- If cross-training, such as water running, does not aggravate the problem, you can maintain conditioning by doing some, at least every other day.

Preventing Injury

Having had over a hundred injuries myself, and then having worked with tens of thousands who have worked through aches and pains, I've developed the suggestions below. They are based upon my experience and are offered as one exerciser to another. I'm proud to report that since I started following the advice that I give others, I've not had an overuse injury in over 30 years.

Take 48 hours between strenuous workouts.
Exercising longer or faster (for you), puts a lot more stress on the muscles tendons. Allowing tired muscles to rest for two days can work magic in recovery. Stair machine work should also be avoided during the 48-hour rest period (stair work uses the same muscles as running). Also avoid any other activities that seem to irritate the aggravated area.

Don't stretch!
I've come full circle on this. A high percentage of the exercisers who report to me, injured, have either become injured because they stretched or aggravated the injury by stretching. When they stop stretching, most have reported that the injury starts healing, in a relatively short period of time. The exception to this rule is in the treatment of iliotibial band injury. For this injury alone, stretching the IT band seems to help runners continue when the band tightens up.

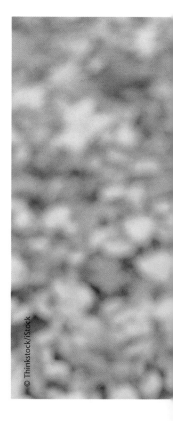

© Thinkstock/iStock

Do the "toe squincher" exercise (prevention of foot and heel injuries).
This exercise can be done 10-30 times a day, on both feet (one at a time). Point the toes and squinch them until the foot cramps (only a few seconds). This strengthens the many little muscles in the foot that can provide a platform of support. It is particularly effective in preventing plantar fascia.

Don't increase total mileage or minutes more than 10% a week more than two weeks in a row.

Monitor your quantity of exercise with a log book or calendar. If you exceed the 10% increase rule, take an extra day off.

Drop total mileage in half, every 3rd or 4th week—even when increasing by no more than 10% per week.

Your log book can guide you here also. You won't lose any conditioning, and you'll help the body heal itself, and get stronger. A steady increase, week after week, does not allow the legs to catch up and rebuild.

Avoid a long stride—whether walking or running.

Use more of a shuffle motion (feet close to the ground), and you'll reduce the chance of many injuries.

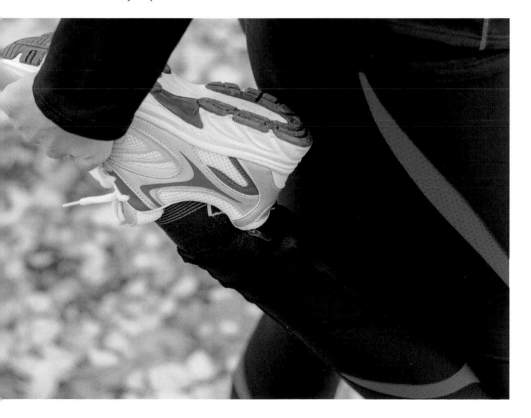

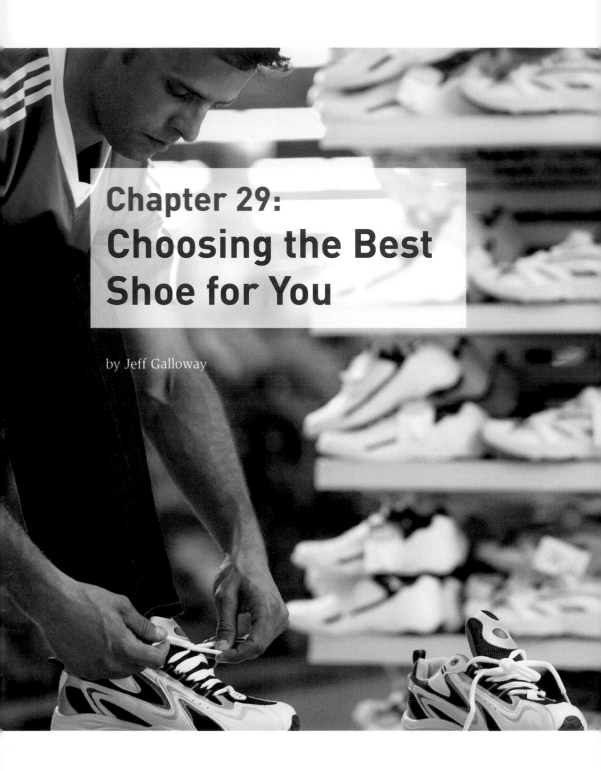

Chapter 29:
Choosing the Best Shoe for You

by Jeff Galloway

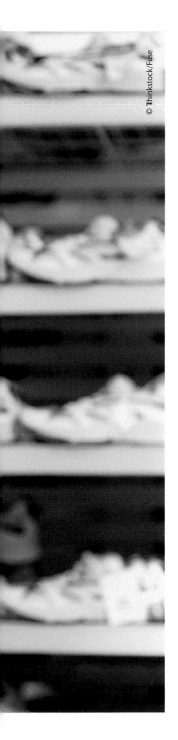

© Thinkstock/Fuse

If you have a good technical running store in your area, go there to get help in fitting. The advice you can receive from experienced shoe fitters will be priceless. My store, Phidippides, has some information on the website www.Phidippides.com. Here are some other helpful tips:

1. Look at the wear pattern on your most worn pair of walking or running shoes. Use this guide to help you choose about three pairs of shoes from one of the categories:

*Flexible?
If you have the wear pattern of a "floppy" or flexible foot, on the inside of the forefoot, and have some foot or knee pain, look at a neutral shoe that does not have a lot of cushion in the forefoot.

*Flexible—Overpronated Foot?
The wear pattern shows significant wear on the inside of the forefoot. If there is knee or hip pain, look for a shoe that has structure or anti-pronation capabilities. If you don't have pain, look at a neutral shoe what does not have a lot of cushion in the forefoot.

*Rigid?
If you have a wear pattern on the outside of the forefoot of the shoe and no wear on the inside, you probably have a rigid foot, and can choose a neutral shoe that has adequate cushion and flexibility for you, as you run and walk in them.

---

*Can't tell?
Choose shoes that are neutral or mid-range of cushion and support.

- Set aside at least 30 minutes to choose your next shoe.
- Run and walk, on a pavement surface, to compare the shoes. If you have a floppy foot, make sure that you get the support you need.
- You want a shoe that feels natural on your foot—no pressure or aggravation—while allowing the foot to go through the range of motion needed for running.
- Again, take as much time as you need before deciding.
- If the store doesn't let you run in the shoe, go to another store.

---

2. Go by fit and not the size noted on the box of the shoe.

Most runners wear a running shoe that is about two sizes larger than their street shoe. For example, I wear a size 10 street shoe but run in a size 12 running model. Be open to getting the best fit—regardless of what size you see on the running shoe box.

3. Include extra room for your toes.

Your foot tends to swell during the day, so it's best to fit your shoes after noontime. Be sure to stand up in the shoe during the fitting process to measure how much extra room you have in the toe region of the shoe. Pay attention to the longest of your feet, and leave at least half an inch.

On race day: Racing shoe or lightweight training shoe?

Most of the high performance racing shoes will lose their cushioning and bounce by the 20-mile mark in a marathon. Most of the runners I've followed who have tried both types of shoes have had better success with a lightweight training shoe. Start breaking in your race shoe about two months prior to race day, by wearing them one day a week for two miles on an easy run. It's also recommended that you wear them during three- to four-mile repeats, during your last two-mile repeat workouts.

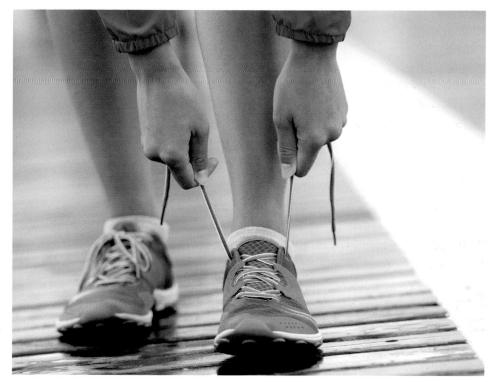

© Thinkstock/iStock

Width Issues

- Running shoes tend to be a bit wider than street shoes.
- Usually, the lacing can "snug up" the difference, if your foot is a bit narrower.
- The shoe shouldn't be laced too tightly around your foot because the foot swells during running and walking. On hot days, the average runner will move up one-half shoe size.
- In general, running shoes are designed to handle a certain amount of "looseness." But if you are getting blisters when wearing a loose shoe, tighten the laces.
- Several shoe companies have some shoes in widths.
- The shoe is too narrow if you are rolling off the edge of the shoe as you push off—on either side.

Shoes for Women

Women's shoes tend to be slightly narrower than those for men, and the heel is usually a bit smaller. The quality of the major running shoe brands is equal whether for men or women. But about 25% of women runners have feet that can fit better into men's shoes. Usually the confusion comes when women wear large sizes. The better running stores can help you make a choice in this area.

Breaking in a New Shoe

- Wear the new shoe around the house, for an hour or more each day for a week. If you stay on carpet, and the shoe doesn't fit correctly, you can exchange it at the store. But if you have put some wear or dirt on the shoe, few stores will take it back.
- In most cases you will find that the shoe feels comfortable enough to run immediately. It is best to continue walking in the shoe, gradually allowing the foot to accommodate to the arch, the heel, the ankle pads, and to make other adjustments. If you run in the shoe too soon, blisters are often the result.
- If there are no rubbing issues on the foot when walking, you could walk in the new shoe for a gradually increasing amount, about two to four days.
- On the first run, just run about half a mile in the shoe. Put on your old shoes and continue the run.
- On each successive run, increase the distance run in the new shoe for three to four runs. At this point, you will usually have the new shoe broken in.

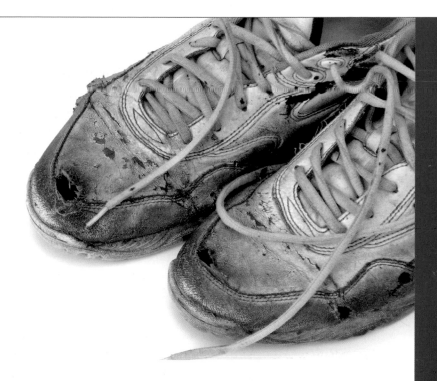

How do you know when it's time to geht a new shoe?

1. When you have been using a shoe for three to four weeks successfully, buy another pair of exactly the same model, make, size. The reason for this: The shoe companies often make significant changes or discontinue shoe models (even successful ones) every six to eight months.
2. Walk around the house in the new shoe for a few days.
3. After the shoe feels broken in, run the first half mile of one of your weekly runs in the new shoe, then put on the shoe that is already broken in.
4. On the "shoe break-in" day, gradually run a little more in the new shoe. Continue to do this only one day a week.
5. Several weeks later you will notice that the new shoe offers more bounce than the old one.
6. When the old shoe doesn't offer the support you need, shift to the new pair.
7. Start breaking in a third pair.

Index

A

B

C

D

E

F

H

I

J

L

S

T

V

W

Credits

Cover design:	Sabine Groten
Cover photo:	© Thinkstock/Stockbyte
Layout and typesetting:	Kerstin Quadflieg
Copy editing:	Elizabeth Evans
Photos:	See individual photos

HILLSBORO PUBLIC LIBRARIES
Hillsboro, OR
Member of Washington County
COOPERATIVE LIBRARY SERVICES